Evaluating the Impact of Health Programs

Evaluating the Impact of Health Programs

A Primer

Michael E. Borus

C. Gregory Buntz

William R. Tash

The MIT Press
Cambridge, Massachusetts
London, England

Publisher's Note

This format is intended to reduce the cost of publishing
certain works in book form and to shorten the gap between
editorial preparation and final publication. Detailed
editing and composition have been avoided by photographing
the text of this book directly from the authors' camera-
ready copy.

Printed and bound in the United States of America

Library of Congress Cataloging in Publication Data

Borus, Michael E.
   Evaluating the impact of health programs.

   Bibliography: p.
   1. Community health services--Evaluation.
2. Ambulatory medical care--Evaluation.
3. Community health services--United States--
Evaluation. I. Tash, William R. II. Buntz, C.
Gregory. III. Title.
RA427.B77   362.1   82-13
ISBN 0-262-52075-3 (pbk.) AACR2

Evaluation in the health field has had a relatively
long history. Nearly 150 years ago a French statisti-
cian and physician, Dr. Pierre Ch. A. Louis, coaxed
his colleagues to "demonstrate, rigorously, the influence and the degree of influence of any therapeutic
agent on the duration, progress, and termination of a
particular disease."[1] Demonstrating the effectiveness
of medical care was an ideal gradually followed by
others. In the late 1850s Florence Nightingale conducted a number of studies evaluating the efficacy of
hospital care of British Army casualties during the
Crimean War. Using such indicators as the number of
hospital deaths per diagnostic category to document
the poor conditions in army hospitals, Nightingale
asserted that changes in sanitation could result in
substantial decreases in care-fatality rates.[2]

In the beginning of the 20th century, Dr. Edward M.
Codman attempted to institute a follow-up system for
the purpose of monitoring patient outcomes at Massachusetts General Hospital. The system was designed to
examine all patients for post operative progress.
Unfortunately, Dr. Codman's ideas on evaluation at
that time were too advanced for the Massachusetts
General administration to adopt, and Codman had to
wait several years before implementing the system at a
private institution which he himself founded.

The medical community's interest was centered more
at this time on issues surrounding the licensing and
training of physicians than the assessment of the
outcomes of medical care. The Flexner Report,
published in 1910, for example, called for major
changes in the structure and organization of medical
education. The report advised medical institutions to
do away with poorly prepared and unlicensed medical
practitioners. The report, however, gave little
attention to the assessment of the medical care provided, or the outcomes of care.

---

[1]Quoted in Christoffel and Loventhal (36), p. 877.

[2]Quoted in Brock and Avery (24).

The College of Surgeons shortly afterwards under-
took a survey of nearly 700 hospitals and concluded
that few institutions were equipped to provide a
minimum level of quality care to patients. In 1919
the College instituted a program of minimum standards
for all hospitals to follow. Eventually this program
evolved into the accreditation process employed by the
Joint Commission on Accreditation of Hospitals (JCAH)
which was founded in 1951.

During World War II and throughout the post-war
period evaluators of medical care shifted attention
from standard setting to a review of the care giving
process. Information about what was happening to
patients, rather than the qualifications of the care
givers, became the key consideration. The medical
audit of the patient's record, rather than the certification of the institutional process, became central
to the new technology which emerged to support the
evaluation process.

The basic assumption underlying the use of the
medical audit was that information on the patient's
chart reflected the actual performance of the medical
team. While the shift in emphasis to the care giving
process was an important one, the use of the medical
record alone to support the process proved to be a
major obstacle. Medical evaluators soon discovered
that the data provided by the audit process was often
an inadequate basis for decision making.

With the passage of the 1972 Amendments to the
Social Security Act (P.L. 92-603), the Professional
Standards Review Organization program (PSRO) was
officially mandated to monitor the quality of care
provided at the regional and local levels. While the
medical audit remained a key component of the PSRO
review process, a variety of new evaluation techniques
emerged to complement and strengthen this approach.
Patients were certified for admission based on information collected on patients prior to hospitalization;
a concurrent as well as retrospective review process
was installed at all facilities which were receiving
Medicare and Medicaid funds. The review process also
emphasized the appropriateness, as well as the quality
of the care provided. Throughout the process, evalua-

tors were encouraged to utilize explicit review criteria based on quantitative data.

The evaluation process itself became more formalized as the peer review committee developed into the control element for judging the quality and appropriateness of medical care. Increasingly medical facilities came under the review of outside evaluators and review committees sponsored by third party payors, as well as federal, state, and private accreditation bodies.

During the 1970s and early 1980s there was also renewed interest in the assessment of the outcomes of medical care as earlier advocated by Dr. Codman and Florence Nightingale. A variety of studies incorporated the use of sophisticated outcome measures based on such concepts as the patient's health status, level of functioning, and severity of the disability. Williamson, for example, in the Health Accounting Project assessed both the diagnostic and therapeutic outcomes of care (155).[3] Shapiro's study of the Health Insurance Program of Greater New York's group practice system compared infant mortality rates of HIP subscribers with the general population. Outcome was defined as "some measurable aspect of health status influenced by a particular element or array of those elements of medical care" (127). Kane, et al., developed a method for determining the functional outcome status of patients in an ambulatory setting. The health status of patients was compared at three points in time: usual status, status at the initial visit, and status at time of telephone follow-up after care (88).

More recently interest has shifted to reviewing the outcomes of health care in relation to costs. In 1975, the major portion of an issue of the New England Journal of Medicine was devoted to a discussion of cost benefit analysis. Two years later, another issue

---

[3]Therapeutic outcomes were assessed by predicting the percentage of patients treated which fall into several categories of functional impairment.

of the New England Journal of Medicine included
further discussion and a sophisticated application in
relation to the management of hypertension (151).
Many observers consider these articles, and the volume
by Weinstein and Stason (152), to be landmarks in the
application of cost effectiveness analysis in the
health field.

Recent years have reflected significant growth in
the number of articles in the health care cost benefit
and effectiveness literature. Since 1970 the number of
publications were never less than 25 (132). Clearly,
the rate of growth of these studies vastly exceeds
that of the medical literature in general. Yet, the
above analysis of the existing literature points to
several major shortcomings and gaps in the present
state of the art. Among the shortcomings are:
failure to consider how environmental factors might
alter program inputs and outputs; failure to account
for program effects which might vary in relation to
the size of the program; ignoring increases over time
in the efficiency of a program's operation; the
problem of using "proxy" goals and measures to
estimate program effects and benefits; the problem of
uncertainty about the future, and how to estimate
long-term benefits.

One of the concerns we have had in developing the
ideas for this volume was to provide an evaluation
approach which focused on the diverse processes,
structures, and impacts of health programs in the
context of costs. We felt that looking at the health
inputs, structures, standards of practices, outcomes,
or even costs in isolation would not lead to a comprehensive view of a health program's cost effectiveness. While we recognize that the relationships
between impacts, structure, and processes of care are
far from clear, the attempt to make the connections
can lead to a better understanding of the health
program.

It is our position, therefore, that impact analysis
can be applied even in situations where the benefits
are not precisely known, nor the monetary value of the
benefits agreed upon by various decision makers. Yet,
as Hellinger points out, "the relevant question is not

whether the costs and benefits of various projects can
be measured precisely," but "whether decisions regard-
ing which projects are to be funded should be made
using information on the perceived costs and benefits
of each project."[4]

In the approach proposed in this volume we recognize that the specification of relevant health costs
and impacts depends to a great extent on the values of
the health officials, the public, the government
officials, and the consumer about health and health
care. For this reason we are proposing an approach
which identifies as many health impacts as possible
and allows the various users to set their own priorities in the decision-making process.

We also wish to point out that with decreasing
federal support for health and health-related social
programs, it is becoming increasingly incumbent on
state, city, and county officials to make decisions
about the continuance of public health programs and
services in their jurisdictions. It is our belief,
therefore, that such decisions should be made in the
context of sound evaluation data. Decision makers
also should be able to compare the cost and benefits
anticipated from health investments in relation to
those anticipated from other types of public investments, such as for highway construction, employment
programs, and economic development efforts. This
volume, therefore, suggests a methodology which allows
for the translating of many health benefits into
monetary values which will contribute toward such
comparisons.

Finally, we wish to remind the reader that while
this volume is program focused, much of the methodology discussed is also appropriate for the assessment
of medical interventions or technologies as well as
health programs. We have chosen the health program to
be the primary concern of this volume, however, since
it represents the administrative facility and planning
unit at the community level through which most public

----

[4]Hellinger (78), pp. 205.

ambulatory health care services are provided in this
country.   While there remains considerable confusion
in the literature between health program evaluation
and the assessment of medical interventions, we hold
that sharp lines need not be drawn between the two at
the present time.   Future research endeavors may well
be directed toward amplifying distinctions and providing evaluation approaches most suited to the assessment of new and emerging health technologies.

We wish to acknowledge the support and inspiration of
Robert Walkington, the Director of Evaluation, Health
Resources Administration, HHS, for encouragement in
the planning, development, and execution of this
project.   We wish also to thank Molly Dolan, the
Horizon Institute, for her diligence in typing many
drafts of this volume; Mary Tash, the Horizon
Insitute, for her editing and suggestions on health-
related topics; and Kathi Niehaus and Sherry McNamara
of The Ohio State University for typing of the final
version of the manuscript.

Evaluating the Impact of Health Programs

INTRODUCTION

What is Evaluation?

Evaluation is the systematic gathering of information in order to make choices among alternative courses of action. In terms of health and other social programs, evaluation can be looked upon as the third step in the process of program implementation (see Chart 1.1). The first step is planning. Planning consists of the definition of the health problems to be addressed and the choice of the course of action to be taken in the solution of the problems. The second step is program operations. This is an attempt to solve the problem through the program outlined in the plan. The third step is evaluation which seeks to determine whether the health program was successful in solving the problem or could be more successful than it was.

Obviously, there are links between evaluation and the other two steps in the process. Planning must be based on information gathered in past evaluations. Through the study of the success of past programs we develop better future means to solve our problems because we need not repeat errors made by others, and we can expand those aspects of past programs which have proven to be successful. Similarly, program operations can be altered to maximize the successful elements of the program and to remove or change those

Chart 1.1 The Process of Program Implementation

Planning
Definition of a health problem and the development of a program to solve the problem
Program Operation
An attempt to solve the health program through a specific course of action
Evaluation
Measuring whether the program successfully solved the health problem

facets which are unsuccessful. In this way, evaluation permits us constantly to improve and upgrade the quality and mix of health programs by providing feedback on successes and failures.

Why Evaluate?

One reason for conducting evaluations has just been presented. Humans as thinking, rational animals will seek to choose among alternative courses of action so as to maximize their well being. Systematically gathering information on the success and failure of past actions improves their ability to get the most that they can (maximizes benefits) while giving up as little as necessary (minimizes costs) in present and future actions.

In terms of health programs, however, there are usually other reasons for conducting evaluations, i.e., external pressures and/or requirements to do so. These pressures arise from the relative newness and controversiality of national health programs, especially those directed at health planning and regulation. Health programs also are significant in terms of cost, number of people affected, and in their perceived abilities to do good or harm. Consequently, evaluation of health programs is increasingly required by federal and state legislation.[5] Further, state governments will be called upon to evaluate the effectiveness of various health programs supported by federal block grant funds and local resources. These same factors also have forced program managers to justify the continuation or expansion of their programs to both their superiors and to the public

---

[5]Examples of legislative requirements for evaluation may be found in P.L. 94-63 (Community Mental Health Centers Act) which states that program evaluation must be undertaken and disclosed to residents of a Community Mental Health Center and P.L. 90-490 (Public Health Services Act) which authorizes up to one percent of program funds for evaluation purposes.

through analytical results. Finally, various innovations in public sector budgeting, particularly program budgeting and zero-based budgeting, require a greater analytical justification than was necessary under earlier budgeting systems.

What are the Types of Evaluation?

The evaluation of health programs can be divided into three general types, each of which asks different questions but can be thought of as a continuum of steps to trace out the programs' effects. 1) Process evaluation asks the question, "How did (or does) the program operate?" 2) Impact evaluation asks the question, "What did the program accomplish?" (3) Strategic analysis seeks to answer the question, "How effective was this program in solving specific health problems as compared with all of the other programs directed at the problem?"[6]

Process evaluation compares the manner in which a program is operated and the products it produces against the plan for the program. It is plan oriented--it tests whether the health plan is being carried out as written on the basis that the plan must be

---

[6]This is just one of many taxonomies for describing the types of evaluation. Others may be found in Scriven, whose formative evaluation is similar to process evaluation and summative evaluation roughly corresponds to our impact evaluation (126). Ferman also has an excellent categorization (65). It has also been customary to differentiate between structural and process evaluations in the health field, e.g., structural evaluation involves assessment of the available input resources; and process assessment involves the way the input resources are used. We find, however, the distinction between control and monitoring to be more useful for ambulatory care evaluation, since very few process studies consider only structural inputs.

followed in order to have success.[7] It is operations oriented--it is concerned with what goes on in the program and what the program does to and for the clients.

Process evaluation begins with the assumption that in order to solve a problem certain preconditions must occur.   Therefore, one type of process evaluation (referred to as control evaluation) is to test for the existence of these factors. For example, a federally funded and certified Health Maintenance Organization (HMO) assumes a contractual responsibility to provide or ensure the delivery of a stated range of health services to an enrolled, defined population.   In return, it requires a fixed periodic payment from members that is independent of the use of the HMO's services. A control evaluation would examine the availability of the appropriate resources to meet these obligations. It would examine such elements as the number of health services, e.g., laboratory tests, facilities, medical equipment available.   In fact, HMOs are routinely examined to insure that such services are provided by certified staff.   There is in such evaluations the implicit assumption that in order to receive quality care, professional health staff must meet certain certification requirements and be provided with basic resources to perform their functions.   The control type of process evaluation examines whether the inputs to the program meet a set of predetermined standards.   It also questions if the standards are reasonable.

A second type of process evaluation is monitoring.   The emphasis is still on meeting predetermined standards; however, monitoring focuses on accomplishments or outputs rather than inputs.   A monitoring

---

[7]In the case of program failure, we want to know, "was the idea (the concept) wrong or was it the execution of the idea?" Process evaluation seeks to determine whether the execution was correct, which implies that the plan was inappropriate, or whether the execution was faulty so that the idea was not truly tested.

evaluation asks such questions as "Has the HMO provided adequate preventive services?" or "Is it meeting
the needs of the poor and the aged to the degree
specified in its plan?" or "Is it an efficient user of
allied health personnel and medical technology?"

Impact evaluation seeks to measure the effects of
the program. It tries to answer the question, "What
difference has the program made?" The emphasis is on
the changes brought about by the existence of the
health program. Impact evaluation seeks to compare
what occurs, given the existence of the health program, to what would have occurred if the program did
not exist. For example, impact evaluation seeks to
determine whether persons enrolled in an HMO have less
need for emergency and sick care treatment as compared
to what the treatment level would have been had they
not been enrolled. It is important to note that we
are measuring the changes caused by the HMO intervention. We wish to know not only how much improvement
occurred in the quality of the client's health, but
also whether this was more than would have taken place
were there no HMO.

It should also be noted that impact evaluation
seeks to measure all of the differences caused by the
program and is not limited to only those which were
originally listed as goals for the program in its
plan. It is quite possible that health programs will
have outcomes other than those originally planned.
For instance, an impact evaluation of a family
planning program may measure such diverse impacts
as: numbers of unwanted pregnancies diverted,
increased earnings of clients, reduced costs for
family expenditures, reduced numbers of hospitaliza-
tions for health or mental health care, and improved
scores on quality of life or life satisfaction scales.

Finally, strategic analysis seeks to compare alternative programs in order to judge their relative
efficiency at accomplishing long-run, large-scale
outcomes. Such analysis might compare the relative
merits of providing primary health care through HMOs,
private practice and community health care centers in
terms of improved health care, health status, and life
expectancy. Strategic analysis compares the results

of impact evaluations for more than one program.

In addition to the type of question being asked, another feature which distinguishes the types of evaluation is the time period for which the program is evaluated. Control evaluation examines the structure of the program and its inputs; consequently, it looks at information which is gathered during the involved period of program operation. Monitoring also takes place during the operation of the program but it usually will gather information about post-program results too, or what happens to clients after receiving a specified set of services. Impact evaluation requires a longer period of time after receiving health service to determine the long-run results. Finally, strategic analysis compares the results of impact evaluations from a variety of competing programs and must wait until all of the impact evaluations have been conducted before assessing the results. Strategic analysis is sometimes referred to as metaevaluation in the literature.[8]

The distinctions between the various types of evaluation may be clearer if an example were presented:

1. An administrator evaluates a newly funded and certified HMO to determine if: (a) the required health services are available, (b) the facility is properly staffed by trained and qualified personnel, and (c) clients are not excluded from eligibility on an arbitrary basis. This is control evaluation. It examines inputs to the process and measures them against standards of necessity.

2. As the HMO matures, the administrator periodically measures its operating efficiency to see if patients are receiving the services at the time they would be expected to receive them, whether there are excessive waiting periods for the ser-

---

[8]See Cook, T.D. and Gruder, C.L. (47).

vices, and whether acceptable medical care is
practiced.   This is monitoring.   It examines
progress   and   output   against   predetermined
standards of what should occur.
3. Nursing home patients receive treatment and are
   referred to appropriate hospital care.   The
   administration wishes to measure whether these
   services have reduced morbidity and mortality
   rates.   This is impact evaluation.   It relates
   changes in outputs to a change in the inputs.

4. An evaluator attempts to determine whether it is
   better to support community health centers to meet
   the special health needs of the underserved, or to
   reimburse individual providers for providing such
   health services.   This is strategic analysis.   It
   compares the efficiency of alternative strategies
   for accomplishing a goal.

Who Evaluates?

Types of evaluation may also be differentiated by the
kinds of organizations that conduct them and the uses
to which they are put.   Since control evaluations
basically deal with whether prescribed conditions
exist or do not exist, it is the easiest type of
evaluation to conduct and does not require an intimate
knowledge of the program.   They are usually conducted
by accrediting and standard setting organizations.
This type of evaluation is also associated with the
General Accounting Office (GAO), the "Federal or state
representative" who reviews community programs, and
other "outside" or professional organizations who
attempt to assess and certify programs quickly.   On
the other hand, monitoring usually involves the program managers or members of the program's administrative staff since one of the basic purposes of monitoring is to provide the program administrator with early
feedback on his or her successes and failures.
Monitoring questions are often built into the health
program's management information system to allow for
routine reporting on center operations.
   Impact evaluation is usually done by an external
agency.   Most health program managers do not have the

skills, budget, time, or interest necessary to conduct impact evaluation. Further, internal evaluations may give the appearance of conflict of interest. Hence, contracts for such evaluations are often let by federal, state, or non-profit agencies to private researchers or universities. Finally, strategic analysis can be conducted only at the highest level of decision making since it compares programs and strategies that cut across normal agency and jurisdictional lines. For instance, in the Health and Human Services Administration, the Office of the Assistant Secretary for Health, and the Office of Planning and Evaluation perform the function. In Congress, the House and Senate Budget Committees are responsible for allocating funds across broad subject areas, while the Appropriations Committees divide the funds among competing programs. The Congressional Budget Office (CBO) is charged with providing the analyses on which these decisions are made.[9]

What are Health Programs?

Health programs are single or multi-focused ambulatory health care organizations for the planning and delivery of preventive and health care services at the community level. They may be comprehensive delivery programs such as community health centers, community mental health centers, or health maintenance organizations aimed at maintaining the health of a broad client or constituent group, or relatively single-

---

[9]The types of evaluation are obviously not mutually exclusive. As noted earlier, in the case of a failure (based on an impact evaluation) we want to know whether it is the theory behind the intervention or medical practice or its execution which was faulty (which requires process evaluation). If we have a success (again using an impact evaluation), we will want to make sure that the success was due to interventions being followed and not to some deviations in the procedure.

focused organizations such as family planning clinics, renal dialysis centers, or alcohol treatment clinics aimed at treating and ameliorating specific health conditions for a defined client group.

It is recognized that the boundary lines between comprehensive and single-focused programs are not always clear, and the impacts of such programs may overlap. Family planning programs, for example, may provide fertility and contraceptive services, but also screen clients for sexually transmitted diseases and provide nutritional counseling of parents and screening of infants for childhood disease. Comprehensive health programs may also provide family planning services and other types of specialty services. Yet, the distinction is useful, and provides evaluators assistance in defining priorities among the goals and objectives of these various types of programs.

Health programs differ from various types of medical interventions, which may be provided through the health program, medical service, private physician, or hospital. A medical intervention refers to a medical technology or approach for ameliorating a specific health condition. Health programs, in contrast to health interventions, involve a facility-based organization which undertakes the health care planning and health care delivery for a group of clients. Health programs include the health administration and support staff which collectively plan for the health care of the client population.

The assessment of health technology or interventions may be part of program evaluation, or distinct from program evaluation. As part of program evaluation, questions need to be raised not only if the intervention is successful, but if it is successful within the context of a publicly funded program. Questions also need to be raised relative to the success of the intervention in contrast to other completely different approaches of health care and prevention activity which may be provided by the health program, questions, for example, as to the effectiveness of an application of health technology in contrast to a program of preventive health care for treating specific types of health conditions.

Organization of this Primer

The focus of this primer is on publically supported health programs which are designed to develop health resources or to deliver comprehensive or specialized ambulatory health services to underserved or special populations. These include alcohol and drug abuse, mental health, migrant, community health, Health Maintenance Organizations, family planning, maternal and child health programs. While the material and approach is especially oriented to preventive health, health education, and psycho-social health related programs, it is applicable to many other types of conventional health programs as well.

Further, in this primer we are primarily concerned with impact evaluation. We shall not cover strategic analysis since our purpose is to introduce the reader to the basics of evaluation techniques. In addition, we have decided to concentrate on questions dealing with the mechanics of conducting evaluations and to omit most of the theoretical discussions which have occurred in the field of evaluation (although references to these discussions are provided). We feel that while the techniques for evaluating health programs are not particularly difficult, most past evaluations have not included all of those basic components necessary to arrive at reliable policy decisions. Therefore, we decided to give special emphasis in this monograph to the areas where past studies have failed.

We feel that readers can best use this primer if they attempt to test their knowledge and make use of it as they go along. Therefore, we have included exercises at the end of each chapter. We also suggest that readers examine several of the studies cited in each section. Each of these was selected because it presented theoretical arguments in greater detail than we were able to do in the short space of this primer. Hopefully, this primer, together with the exercises and references, will serve as a jumping-off point in the evaluative process, permitting evaluators to develop their own analyses without committing the same mistakes that have marred earlier studies.

Chapter Outline

The purpose of evaluation is to provide policy makers
and health program managers with the basic data necessary for them to make decisions wisely.   Impact
evaluations of health programs examine the long-run
outcomes of programs and view success and failure in
these terms. They should provide five essential sets
of information.   First, they should provide the data
necessary to determine if a particular health program
should be continued.   Second, they should determine
which of alternative programs achieve the greatest
gains for a given cost.   Third, evaluations should
present information on the components of each program
and the mixes of components which are most effective
for a given expenditure so that maximum operating
efficiency can be achieved.   Fourth, evaluations
should provide the first three types of information
for persons with different characteristics so that a
decision maker may determine which individuals are
best served by each program.   Finally, in the course
of evaluating existing programs, data should be
gathered which will suggest new methods for providing
health care delivery.   Few impact evaluations of
health programs have provided all of this information
to date.
    One of the major problems in the evaluation of
health programs is that they encompass a wide variety
of desired outcomes for the nation's population.
Generally, health programs seek to improve the health
status of the program clients, and in this way, to
better their physical, mental and economic well
being. These goals, however, are broad and difficult
to operationalize. As a consequence, evaluations of
health programs often have been narrow in focus,
usually limited to the most obvious effects of client
care, e.g., the manner in which certain health problems are handled by clinical staff, administrative
support staff, etc. Other less apparent but possibly
important impacts have been frequently ignored.
Therefore, our first task in Chapter 2 is to define
more of the basic objectives and impacts of health
programs and attempt to establish   relevant measurable

critiera.

Other problems which have arisen in health impact evaluations revolve around the question, "Whom do health programs affect?" It appears that past studies have often excluded, either because of a lack of data or a theoretical bias, many persons whose experiences were influenced by such programs. In Chapter 2, we point out some of the other groups that also should be examined.

The designs for measuring the success of health programs in past studies have often been weak. Many of the problems have arisen in the use of control or comparison groups. To estimate the effects of a program, it is necessary to compare the experience of the program clients with that of some reference group whose experience can be said to represent what would have happened to the clients in the absence of the program. Unfortunately, results of past studies, which were contrary to the prejudices of policy makers, have been dismissed too often on the grounds of noncomparability between program clients and "controls." In Chapter 3, we present a procedure which we feel will best solve the comparability problems. We also supply descriptive information on possible sources of data which might be useful for measuring the benefits of health programs.

The problems involved in measuring the costs of health programs have been similar to those involved in measuring program success. Past studies often have not measured all of the appropriate costs, have inadequately selected control groups for cost analysis, and have ignored some groups who incur costs. These are the issues discussed in Chapter 4.

A final problem which has limited the usefulness of many previous evaluations has been the lack of comparability in the presentation of the results of these studies. In Chapter 5, therefore, we present a suggested schema for comparing program benefits and costs. We suggest ways to place monetary value on various health benefits. We also suggest in that chapter a number of technical aspects which have often been lacking in prevoius studies--the of multivariate analysis to separate the influences of the wide variety of possible determinants of program success, the use of marginal analysis whenever possible, and the methods for projecting and discounting future effects of the programs. In Chapter 5 we also present a summary outline of the procedural steps which we have discussed in earlier chapters.

Exercise 1-1

Label each of the following types of evaluation questions as control, monitoring, impact, or strategic
analysis.

1. Do all staff of a community health center have
   proper certification for the activities they are
   performing?
2. Does a health maintenance organization provide all
   the contracted services to its enrolled population?
3. Do the clients who participate in nutritional
   education classes actually practice better dietary
   habits after a six-month or year period?
4. Is the average waiting time per encounter for
   scheduled visits at a health clinic realistic?
5. Are the number of days lost from work for health
   or mental health reasons reduced for members of an
   HMO?
6. Do clients who utilize mental health services
   reduce their utilization rates for other types of
   health services?
7. Do economic incentives provide a better mechanism
   for increasing the distribution of physicians to
   rural areas than legislative regulations?
8. Are the costs for HMO enrollees growing less
   rapidly than costs in the overall medical care
   sector?

Exercise 1-2

Given the reduced availability of funds for the support of public health programs, what types of
agencies/officials will need to become more deeply
involved in the evaluation of health programs in the
future?

Suggested Readings

Attkisson, C., Hargreaves, W.A. and Horowitz, M.J., eds. Evaluation of Human Service Programs, New York: Academic Press, 1978.

Congress of the United States, Office of Technology Assessment, The Implications of Cost-Effectiveness Analysis of Medical Technology, "Background Paper #1: Methodological Issues and Literature Review," September, 1980.

Cook, T.D. and Gruder, C.L. "Metoevaluation Research, Evaluation Quarterly, 1978, 2, pp. 5-51.

Drummond, M.F. Principles of Economic Appraisal in Health Care, Oxford University Press, 1972.

Layard, R., ed. Cost Benefit Analysis, Middlesex, England: Penguin Books, 1977.

Mishan, E.J. Cost Benefit Analysis, Washington, D.C.: Praeger Publication, 1976.

Riechen, H.W., and Boruch, R.F., ed. Social Experimentation, New York: Academic Press, 1974.

Schulberg, H.C. Program Evaluation in the Health Fields, New York: Behavioral Publications, Inc., 1969.

Struening, E. and Guttentag, M., eds. Handbook of Evaluation Research, Vol. 1, Beverly Hills: Sage Publications, 1975.

THE IMPACT OF HEALTH PROGRAMS

Defining the Goals and Impacts of Health Programs

Health programs may affect many persons and institutions in a variety of ways. Some of these are direct
benefits which are planned. We define those effects
which are objectives of the program planners or
managers as "program goals". There usually are many
other possible effects of these programs which are not
anticipated in the program either because they are
side effects or occur to persons who are not directly
involved in the program. Some of these are positive
outcomes; others may do harm. These unanticipated
effects, along with the goals, we call "impacts".
Thus, program goals are a subset of the program's
impacts.

In our opinion an attempt should be made to measure
all of the impacts and not just the goals. Rationale
for this opinion appears below.

Final Versus Intermediate Outcomes as Impacts

In considering impacts it is useful to distinguish
between the ultimate impacts and those which are only
intermediate steps to achieving those objectives. For
instance, quality-adjusted life years saved may be the
ultimate goal or benefit for participants of an HMO,
but accessible, available and quality services are the
necessary steps to achieve these final outcomes.

Sometimes evaluations must focus on intermediate
outcomes. Intermediate outcomes can be differentiated
in two respects: they occur sooner and/or they are
only partial measures of the ultimate health
impacts. They are usually necessitated by an in-
ability to define adequately the final outcomes, or
not wanting to wait until the final outcomes occur.
(Many health technologies, for example, can be only
evaluated in terms of such intermediate outcomes as
blood counts per minute, or clarity of the X-ray
film.) There is a danger, however, that early results
may not be indicative of longer term consequences.

There are also various types of longer range benefits which may be overlooked.

More seriously, intermediate outcomes may not measure the same factors as the ultimate outcomes. For instance, lower rates of hospitalization for HMO enrollees may not correlate with life years saved. Likewise, person may reduce dependence on drugs, but substitute other forms of deviancy that lead to more negative outcomes. In these cases the implicit assumption that the intermediate outcomes are identical or highly correlated with the ultimate objective is incorrect.

For these reasons it is useful to define impacts in terms of ultimate objectives whenever possible. Similarly, care should be taken when establishing measurement criteria to use those which most closely reflect the ultimate objectives. The further removed that which is being measured is from the eventual outcome in concept and time, the greater the chance of inadequate or improper estimates of the true impacts.

Sources of Impact Definitions

The first order of business in conducting an impact evaluation is to define the broad impacts and the more specific criteria which may be used to judge the effectiveness of the programs.[10]   Where do we find these impacts and criteria?

The obvious place to begin is with the goals as defined in the legislation of established programs to see what the drafters thought the program would accomplish. Unfortunately, this will very often lead to statements that are difficult to operationalize with measurable criteria. For instance, the Health Planning and Resources Development Act of 1974 (P.L. 93-641) has the following Statement of Purpose: "to

---

[10]See, National Center for Health Statistics (106) for a valuable source of reports on measures, evaluations, and impacts of health service programs.

facilitate the development of recommendations for a
national health planning policy to augment areawide
and state planning for health services, manpower and
facilities and to authorize financial assistance for
the development of resources to further that
policy." The statement alludes to the expected short
range outputs (recommendations for a national health
planning policy) and inputs (financial assistance for
the development of resources to further that policy)
but lacks precision as to the structure by which it
will be accomplished, and the specific objectives, and
criteria by which it will be judged. Legislative
language is notoriously vague as a review of a few
other pieces of legislation will show.

Other sources of information on potential impacts
are the legislative hearings held prior to the establishment of the program and the hearings held on
appropriations. Again, however, one is usually left
with vague statements of overall objectives. Moreover, the goals of a program may change over time from
those originally stated in the legislative process.
For instance, the Community Mental Health Center Act
of 1964 was originally intended to demonstrate the
effectiveness of community based mental health treatment. Some now argue that the program's present
purpose is to support the nationwide deinstitutionali-
zation of mental health care. As recent examinations
of U.S. mental health policy show, these are not
necessarily complementary goals.

One can also turn to the managers of the program,
program clients, and other potential users of the
evaluation to obtain their perceptions of the
program's goals. It is important to note, however,
that the goals of program clients will be highly
individualized and will probably be limited to their
personal desires. Likewise, program managers will
often think more about the services which they must
provide and the techniques for delivery than about the
impacts of providing services. Therefore, the suggestions both groups offer are often incomplete and
narrow in their viewpoint.

The organization funding the evaluation also may
offer recommendations on which potential impacts

focus. A problem with relying on the funding organization to define the objectives to be studied is the
possibility of being co-opted. Scriven (126) argues
for "goal-free evaluation" where the evaluator selects
the criteria for evaluating a program independent of
the program staff. Such independence, however, may
cause the evaluator to overlook relevant goals and
criteria. Knowing the goals of the staff need not
necessarily bias the evaluator.

Since these sources of goals are limited in their
ability to supply the evaluator with all of the potential impacts to be examined, it is incumbent on him or
her to think of all the possible areas in which the
program could conceivably have an effect. That many
of these will not be stated objectives for the program
is not important. For example, there is nothing in
the health planning legislation which addresses the
program's effects on the labor market experience of
health care consumers. Yet, P.L. 93-641 may have
impacts in this area because health status and earnings and employment are closely related; to the extent
that health planning improves the health status of a
population, then, their labor market experience may
also improve. Thus, while employment and earnings
were not mentioned by the authors of the Act, they
might be very much affected by health planning. The
impact in this area may be considered very important
by some people using the program's evaluations for
decision making.

As a general rule, it is much better to attempt to
measure impacts which prove not to exist than to
ignore impacts which do exist. There are two reasons
for this. First, both the political and economic
scene may change as time passes, and the goals of the
program may change (as was seen with the Community
Mental Health Centers Act of 1964). If new goals are
not included in an evaluation, it may be worthless
since it will not answer the questions being asked
under the new conditions. Second, since models of the
effects of health care delivery are very incomplete,
they are unable to predict with certainty where the
impact of various health programs will be felt.
Health professionals are unable to model all of the

relationships or to state unequivocally what the
effect of a particular action will be.   As more and
more evaluations are conducted and as a wider variety
of possible impacts are examined, the state of the art
will undoubtedly improve.

     Thus, while it is valuable to determine who will be
using the evaluation and what its uses are to be,
getting complete insights on the success of the programs under evaluation usually makes it imperative to
go beyond these considerations and to include all of
the possible impacts.   Great care should be taken
before an objective is eliminated from consideration
due to the particular uses for which the evaluation is
purported to be made.   A change in the political party
or the economic situation may drastically change the
value   structure   used   to   rank   the   alternative
impacts.   The evaluator must remember that, while it
is   always   possible   to   disregard   information   once
collected, if an impact has been omitted entirely from
the study, it will require an entirely new evaluation
to test for its effects.

Defining Whose Impacts Will be Measured

In   establishing   the   benefits   to   be   studied   it   is
extremely   important   to   note   that   programs   affect
different   groups   in   different   ways   and   at   different
levels.   We can identify four primary parties who may
benefit from health programs.   These are society as a
whole,   program   participants,   health   agencies   and
professionals, and the government.   Each of the groups
has different goals which they wish the health program
to accomplish.   Therefore, depending on the perspective   taken,   the   objectives   of   the   program   will
differ.   From a societal point of view the goals of
health   programs   are   put   in   terms   of   aggregate
changes.   Examples of societal goals would be improved
health status of the population, improved equity in
the   overall   distribution   of   health   services,   and
increased national production.   For the individual
participant the goals are more usually limited to
direct benefits such as a more healthful life or
increased satisfaction with life. Health professionals

too, will tend to look at the programs in terms of their own interests. For instance, the health professionals will be concerned with the quality of care provided, income which results to them for providing the care, and improvements in the client's overall health. Finally, the government will view the programs in terms of the various societal objectives but, in addition, will seek programs which will aid its budgetary position by increasing revenues and reducing expenditures.

Obviously, there is a great deal of overlap among the goals of the various groups. The government acts as the agent of society in operating the programs. As such, definitions of program success will coincide in most areas for the government and for society. Similarly, individuals and health professionals as members of society are interested in aggregate as well as direct changes. Likewise, the effect of programs on individuals and health organizations and professionals will determine in part the programs' success in terms of society. The improved health of participants in programs, for example, is likely to improve the aggregate health status of the nation or community.

There also may be an overlap between the goals of each of the parties. For instance, the reduction in an individual's sick days may increase earnings as well as decrease feelings of dependency. Since the effects may have independent importance for the individual, we believe that all should be considered.

There may be conflicts, however, among the goals of the different parties and among various goals for a particular party. Thus, we may find that a program which improves the health of the participants is very costly to the government or that a program which is highly efficient at controlling health care costs leads to greater inequity in the national distribution of health care services. These conflicts of possible program achievements raise the problem of ranking the objectives of each of the parties and of determining which party's goals have precedence. While on a theoretical level one can argue that societal objectives should be paramount, the evaluator must be a realist. He or she should recognize that the rewards

and costs of health programs to particular interested
parties may play an important role in determining the
size, scope, and even the existence of the program.

Likewise, it should be noted that there are other
groups, particularly pressure groups, who may be less
directly affected by health programs but whose benefits also should be considered because of their
political influence. Health programs, because they
are publicly sponsored, must satisfy political demands
as well as accomplish social and economic good. Who
participates in health programs, and who manages
health programs may be as important politically as
what the programs actually accomplish. Thus, the
effects of health programs through their positive or
negative impact upon voters or campaign contributors
may be extremely important to their political
survival.

Even if we ignore these political considerations
(an action which we do not recommend) health programs
can indirectly affect a number of people. For
instance, a community may be able to increase its
efforts on other activities if it can control its
expenditures on health care delivery. Schools will
face a variety of changes if a migrant health program
improves the learning abilities of a number of children. The families of participants may be adversely
affected by the initial costs which they have to bear
to enroll in an HMO but may subsequently benefit if
the program successfully improves their health and
eventual earning capacity. The point is, one should
consider all of the categories of persons who possibly
could be affected by health programs as well as the
many ways in which these programs could have an
impact.[11]

---

[11]Among the various parties to Community Mental Health
Centers are: Congress, NIMH, state governments,
mental health agencies, local governments, third-party
payors, grantees, mental health professionals, recipients of services, the unserved but eligible population, citizens affected by admission of mental

We hasten to add that the determination of which or whose impacts will be measured should not be left solely to evaluators. Indeed, if one expects the results of an evaluation to be utilized, one must weigh heavily the information needs of decision makers. In addition, the politics of public program evaluation dictates that the users as well as the "doers" of evaluation must participate in the selection of impact measures.

Listing of Potential Benefits from Health Programs

To facilitate the choice of impacts to be studied we present lists of potential benefits for society, individuals, health professionals, and the government. We feel that all health-related programs can be judged in terms of these impacts, but simultaneously realize that each program will have a different method of reaching its objectives and will put a somewhat different emphasis on each of them. Further, because it is our belief that the positive results of most health programs will exceed any negative impacts which may occur, our discussion of impacts is stated in terms of benefits here and throughout this book. Finally, the list is obviously not all-inclusive. It should, however, provide many of the most important outcomes of health programs. Below each benefit we present operational criteria to measure program success in meeting the objective. These criteria are presented as examples of the measures which could be used. Again, the list is not meant to be all-inclusive.

A. Benefits for Society
    1. Improved Health Status.
        a. Increased Life Extension; Reduced Mortality and Morbidity Rates; Increased

---

patients into institutions, interest groups including representatives of mental health professionals, consumers of mental health services, and the general public.

Number of Quality-Adjusted Life Years Saved;[12]

b. Increased Number of Days without Illness or Disability; Increased Proportion of Healthy to Unhealthy Days; Reduced Severity of Disease;

c. Increased Number of Days without Social/Psychological Dysfunctioning Due to Alcoholism, Drugs or Mental Illness; Reduced Severity of Mental Illness;

d. Increased Proportions of Inpatients and Chronically Ill who Return to Community Settings from Long Term Health Care Institutions;

e. Reduced Restrictions on Activities and Years of Restriction as Compared to Longer Life Spans (as measured by such scales as the Pulses Functional Profile and Barthel Index);

f. Improved Scores on Health Status Indexes for Mental, Dental, and Physical Health; General Perceptions of People Concerning Their Health;[13]

g. Improved Scores on Annual Indexes of Health;

h. Reduced Incidence and Prevalence of Treatable Communicable Diseases.

2. Improved Equity in the Distribution of Health Services, Especially for Underserved and Special Target Groups.

a. Improved Health Status. Increase in number of quality-adjusted life years saved, number of days without illness, disability and social/psychological

---

[12]See Weinstein and Stason (150), Fein (63), and Layard (96) for a discussion of various types of weighting schemes.

[13]See, "Health Status Indexes" (76), Balinsky and Bergan (10), and Murnaghn (104).

dysfunctioning for target group members relative to other citizens.

    b. Increased Employment and Income. The increase in the income for target group members and the decrease in the percentage of time in which they are unemployed for reasons of health, relative to the average for all workers.

3. Increased National Production. The increase in the Gross National Product (GNP) which should approximate the sum of the changes in earnings of all persons affected by the programs, including persons who are not program participants.

4. Reduced Unemployment. The decline in the average percentage of time in which persons affected by the program, including nonparticipants, are unemployed for reasons of health or mental illness.

5. Increased Social Functioning and Satisfaction.

    a. Increased Social Functioning. The increase in average scores on social functional measures and client perception scales, e.g., Cornell Medical Index, the Heinler Scale of Social Function, the Katz Adjustment Scale.

    b. Increased Satisfaction with Health Institutions. Improvement in average scores on scales of attitudes toward health institutions, such as health, mental health centers, drug and alcohol abuse facilities.

    c. Improved Overall Quality of Life. The improvement in average scores on various quality of life measures, and self-assessed health status measures in reference to psychological and socioeconomic well being, physical well being and disability.

    d. Improved Self Esteem. Through restriction of parts of the body and overall health, and reduction of disability, suffering, emotional problems, and reduced quality of life that often accompanies disease or illness.

6. Reduced Health Care Costs. The reduction in
the rate of increase of health care costs
relative to the increase in the consumer price
index. Reduction in numbers of hospitaliza-
tions and use of costly medical technology and
care.[14]

7. Reduced Antisocial Behavior. The reduction in
the number of persons affected by the program
who are arrested and convicted of crimes, or
reckless driving while under the influence of
alcohol or drugs, or who are involved in other
socially unacceptable activities.

8. Reduced Dependency on Government. The reduction in the number of persons who receive
public assistance and Medicaid, the amount
received of each, and the proportion of time
these are received. Reduction of income spent
on alcohol and drugs. Psychological scales of
dependency might also be used to examine the
degree of dependency as perceived by persons
whom the program affects.

9. Improved Family Life. The reduction in the
proportion of program-affected persons whose
family lives are negatively altered (through
the consequences of disease such as divorce,
widowhood, changes in residence, orphaned).
Measures of client and family distress could
also be used.

10. Reduced Discrimination and Improved Race
Relations. The proportion of persons affected
by the program who improve their behavior
toward persons of another race, ethnic group,
age, and sex because of more equitable health
care services.

11. Improved Housing. The average improvement in
the quality of housing based on the Census
definitions, especially for persons with

---

[14]Overall the cost of health care rose 120% as compared to 95% for all costs between 1969 and 1980 as
measured by the Consumer Price Index.

physical or mental disabilities as a result of
program activities.

B. Benefits for Individuals
   1. Improved Health Status.
      a. Increased Number of Quality-Adjusted Life
          Years Saved.
      b. Increased Number of Days Without Illness
          or Disability; Proportion of Healthy to
          Unhealthy Days.
      c. Increased Number of Days Without
          Social/Psychological Dysfunctioning Due to
          Alcoholism, Drugs, or Mental Illness.
      d. Improved Scores on Health Status Indexes.
   2. Increased Income. The average increase in the
       disposable income of participants. The
       increase could be from either increased
       employment, higher levels of productivity, or
       reduced expenditures for health care premiums
       and out-of-pockect health costs. Separate
       calculations may be made for various groups of
       participants, e.g., former alcoholics, chroni-
       cally ill, etc.
   3. Reduced Unemployment. For various types of
       program participants (particularly the chroni-
       cally ill), the reduction in the average
       percentage of the time since entering the
       program that they are unemployed for reasons
       of health or drinking.
   4. Increased Satisfaction.
      a. Increased Satisfaction with Work. The
          average improvement in scores on job
          satisfaction tests by different types of
          program participants.
      b. Increased Satisfaction with General Condi-
          tions. The increase in average scores on
          social indicators by different types of
          program participants.
   5. Increased Social Status. The improvement in
       social and occupational status of participants
       with differing characteristics as measured by
       socioeconomic scales.
   6. Increased Voluntary Leisure. The increase in

the average number of hours which are devoted to leisure activities.

7. Reduced Dependency. The reduced proportion of different participant groups who receive public assistance and Medicaid, and the reduction in the amount received of each. The reduction in the degree of dependency as perceived by each group could also be examined. Scales of dependency might be used.

8. Improved Family Life. The reduction in the proportion of program-affected persons whose family lives are negatively altered. Changes in attitudes toward other family members could also be examined.

9. Improved Housing. The average increase in quality of housing of program participants with different characteristics based on the Census definitions.

C. Benefits for Health Professionals and Professional Organizations.

1. Improved Public Relations with Community. The proportion of members from various health organizations who report better communication with constituents as a result of the improved care.

2. Improved Ratings and Stature. Increase in ratings relative to quality assurance reviews. Fewer exceptions or deficiencies found in practice of care.

3. Increased Earnings and Reduced Costs. Earnings are increased as a result of lower utilization rates in prepaid medical plans and increased numbers of persons covered.

4. Increased Time for Social and Professional Improvement. As emergency care needs decrease, greater time is available for leisure and professional development.

D. Benefits for Government Operations.

1. Reduced Transfer Payments. The reduction in Medicaid, disability, public assistance, unemployment insurance or other transfer

payments to program participants and their families.

2. Reduced Costs of Government Operations. The reduction in the use of other public health, vocational rehabilitation, substance abuse, mental health and similar services, after participating in the health program. For example, health care services may be reduced as a result of utilization of mental health program services.

3. Increased Tax Revenues Through an Increased Tax Base. The increase in the taxes paid by persons involved with the program. Separate calculations should be made for federal, state, and local taxes.

Discussion of Criteria

The scope, nature, and purposes of publicly supported health programs in the United States varies widely to say the least. Some are largely targeted toward specific types of diseases and population groups; others are comprehensive and open to all enrollees of a defined geographic area. Some focus on preventive or rehabilitative activities and services, while others largely provide client treatment. This list of impacts attempts to be broad enough to relate to these diverse types of programs.

In defining the many impacts of health programs, we recognize that it is difficult to measure many types of impacts in the health area. We also acknowledge that it is sometimes impossible to establish causality between the program or program services and the many impacts described. Yet, we hold that there is great value in describing impacts for clarifying assumptions, relationships, and identifying probable relationships between interventions, programs, and impacts.

The list of benefits exhibits a heavy economic influence. This is due to our assumption that health care expenditures, whether made by government or indivduals, are in fact investments as well as consumption expenditures. They are investments in the physical and mental well being of individuals. They are expected to result in healthier, more satisfied and productive human beings.

We believe that society is willing to support public investments in health care for four reasons. First, the maintenance of high quality health is considered to be a right and of important value for all Americans. Second, as healthier individuals increase their earnings, the income distribution in the society as a whole may be improved. Thirdly, the improvement in the health of the labor force will permit society to produce more and better goods and services. Finally, society appears interested in improving the earnings and employment of certain of its groups because of the belief in the "Protestant Ethic." Society appears intent on replacing welfare with work, placing a positive value on income earned as opposed to income from other sources (at least among the poor). Therefore, as health programs are directed at specific groups which are poor and likely to receive transfer payments, the attainment of higher earnings and employment for the group is looked upon as a benefit of the program.

Impact analysis also seeks sometimes to express the benefits of health programs in monetary terms (even if here, too, there will be substantial disagreement as to how best to do this). A central issue entails placing a value on the three major health effects of programs, i.e. (1) additional years of healthy life or survival resulting from treatment or cure; (2) additional years of survival but with a disability, illness, or care procedure which restricts one's full enjoyment of life; and (3) improvement in health without any effect on survival. While admittedly such value-setting necessarily reflects the values of the evaluator, there are a number of approaches which offer promise of objectivity used to estimate the monetary value of a healthy life for various age and sex groups.[15] Yet, these approaches imply that the

---

[15]Essentially, economists calculate the earnings that

worth of a life is determined solely by productivity. Another approach, suggested in Layard (96),
which overcomes this bias, entails questioning people
as to what value they place on extended life spans
given certain disabilities as compared to healthy life
extensions.

Economic value can also be placed on various types
of disabilities, impairments, and illnesses. It is
based on people's "willingness to pay" for various
types of treatment. For example, a sick person may be
"willing to pay" $50 for a doctor's help but not
$100. One hospital may be willing to pay $100,000 for
a scanning device but not $500,000. The "willingness-
to-pay" approach has been central to the federal
government's decision to pay for kidney dialysis and
heart transplants. Willingness to pay is also at the
center of many disputes between costs and benefits of
an array of health and safety rules. (Such judgments,
for example, are constantly being made by the courts
in insurance cases in regard to accident, impairments,
and illness/disease resulting from negligence.)16

a person can expect to collect over a lifetime, based
on normal life expectancy as well as sex and race.
They plot the point in midlife when a person's maximum
earnings are still ahead. For example, for white men
this is around the ages 30 to 34. Then, working
backward from that point, they assign a present value
to the lifetime earnings for the very young who have
not reached their prime. Also, working from the
midlife point, they take into account the gradual
decline in earnings as the person ages. The result of
this is a chart which estimates what a person is
worth. See Cooper and Rice (49), and Berg (13) for
further discussion.

16Valuation of life by demand revealing processes such
as the willingness-to-pay criterion was judged still
too experimental and not recommended as a substitute
for the human capital methodology as discussed in this
primer by a recent PHS Task Force. See Hodgson and
Meiners (80).

In regard to change in society's production as a
result of improved health we assume it will be equal
to the increment caused by the health program in the
productive ability of the program members. Since it
is difficult to measure productive ability directly,
the evaluator must rely on marginal productivity
theory which says that the increment in the marginal
individual's output is equal to the increment in his
or her wage, assuming perfect competition. Thus, we
can say that health programs increase the output of
society in an amount equal to the increment in the
earnings of the program members.[17]

Other types of economic impacts are the effects on
government receipts and expenditures. Health programs
themselves require government expenditures. On the
other hand, to the extent that they increase the
health and ultimately the earnings of clients, the
programs will increase the income and other taxes that
these individuals pay. Moreover, if these individuals
are presently provided with health services which lead
to higher earnings, future governmental expenditures
on their behalf will be reduced.[18] Hence, there can
be sizeable impacts of health oriented programs on the
government when one views the government as an economic entity which attempts to maximize the returns to
its resources. This is the way that Congress and many
individuals look upon government programs.

There are other economic benefits to society, the
government and the individual. These, however, are
indirect. For instance, to the extent that health

---

[17]One might also consider the effects of the program
expenditures on income distribution. Some people have
claimed that health programs have distributed more to
the middle class than they have to the poor because it
is the middle class who is paid to provide health
services to the poor.

[18]In these terms, government expenditures for
resources and expenditures which take the form of
transfer payments are treated identically.

programs lead to better health they may make for a
more productive labor force. To the extent that
earnings are increased, crime may be reduced thereby
reducing government and societal expenditures for
certain crime prevention and law enforcement
agencies. There may be a reduction in the need for
social services agencies if programs lead to better
family life through increased earnings. Each of these
indirect effects expands the production possibilities
for society by either improving the resources or
reducing the alternative use of resources. The
measurement of these indirect economic effects, however, appears to be out of the scope of most present
studies. This is at least partially the case because
studies only recently began to look at the effects of
health programs on such factors as employment, crime
and family life.

There are many noneconomic benefits which may
result from health programs particularly for the
individuals who participate in the programs. The
argument is often made that these impacts are not
measurable. This is not always true, as some examples
will demonstrate. The possibility of improved health
has already been discussed. There are a wide variety
of possible measures of an individual's health. Some
of these, such as days of disability, provide cardinal
measures of the impact of health programs.

In the case of individual fulfillment, there are a
wide variety of satisfaction and alientaion scales.
There are scales of social satisfaction, job satisfaction, security, and the like. In most cases, these
have at least ordinal ranking and are reliable and
internally consistent. For references to these scales
the reader should refer to the excellent volumes by
Robinson and others (114, 115).

There also are political goals which may be
achieved through health programs. For individuals,
these may include greater exercise of political
power. For elected officials, it may mean reelec-
tion. For society, it may mean maintenance of the
present system by improving the well-being of program
clients and reducing the likelihood of socially
destructive conflict. These benefits would be

measured by determining the change in political behavior of the participants in the programs and the effects of the participants' actions on the political behavior of other persons.

There may also be social benefits as a result of health programs. It may be thought to be socially desirable to reduce illness and disabiity, to reduce unemployment, to get people off welfare, to have a more integrated society, to have more equal opportunity, to reduce poverty, to care for children and the elderly, and to improve social mobility. If these are considered as desirable benefits which may result from the programs, they need to be measured. For instance, to measure the reduction in unemployment we can look at both aggregate and individual levels. Just as earlier the increment in earnings was assumed to equal the increment in total production, we can also assume that at the margin the increase in employment of the individual will equal the increase of employment in the society. Similarly, we can aggregate reductions in Medicaid and welfare payments and the proportion of program participants who are moved off of welfare.

To measure the integrating effects of health programs we can examine changes in housing patterns, and the change in post participation associations. In the area of equality of opportunity, we can examine changes in the outlook of the participants and in their opportunity for employment. In the areas of social mobility, we can look at the correlation between the parents' and the children's socioeconomic status. This is, of course, a long-range impact of health programs, if it even exists.

Issues Relating to the Choice of Health Measures, and the Comparison of Various Outcomes

The earliest cost-benefit studies simply used the concept life-saved, as a single outcome measure, and assumed that decreases in mortality correlated with decreases in morbidity, pain, and suffering. One of the first efforts to modify the use of this single outcome measure was taken by Klarman (91), who

refined the concept to reflect quality. He argued
that a year of life with a well-functioning transplanted kidney was preferred to a year of life in
dialysis. He, consequently, valued life on dialysis
as equal to .75 years with a transplanted kidney.
Yet, such valuations were arbitrary and far from
satisfying. Bush (28) subsequently developed a health
status index producing weights that range from death
to complete health. Another way of dealing with the
problem is using the concept quality-adjusted life
years, as suggested by Klarman (90). This concept
formed the basis for Weinstein and Stason's (150) use
of an index of health effects in their study of hypertension screening and treatment programs. It requires
adding changes in life expectancy to changes in
quality-adjusted life expectancy resulting from reduction in morbidity, and subtracting changes in quality-
adjusted life expectancy due to iatrogenic illness and
treatment involved side effects. This method also
involves selection of appropriate weights for weighting such concepts. One way to avoid final decisions
is to simply identify and present an array of noncom-
parable measures of effects including rank-ordered
ones. Thus, it becomes the problem of the user to
make judgments about the various outcomes.

We prefer to translate outcomes into a monetary
metric wherever possible, but at the same time identify the underlying assumptions for the readers in the
application of the metric. If certain impacts are
still unable to be transferred to a monetary metric,
these outcomes should be displayed, however, for consideration by the users.

The Choice of Impacts and Criteria

Obviously, we believe that all potential impacts
should be measured if possible. There may time or
budgetary constraints, however, which limit the number
of impacts which can be examined. In these cases the
evaluator should use two factors to determine which
impacts to measure--1) the expected magnitude and
importance of the impacts, and 2) the ease and cost of
measurement.

The assignment of priorities to specific impacts must be the ultimate responsibility of the decision maker to whom the evaluation will be delivered; that person should decide the relative importance of the measured impacts. One can argue, however, that certain impacts, such as those on the health status of participants, must be included in those presented to the decision maker. On the other hand, it may be argued that some impacts are likely to be so small that they are the best candidates for elimination if some impacts must be ignored. For instance, for certain health programs the proportion of the participants who will have been convicted of a crime or even arrested may be so small that any impact on these variables must be negligible. In this situation the omission of the antisocial behavior impact would seem justified if there were severe resource limitations and the collection of arrest data were costly. On the other hand, if the program consisted of providing mental health services to drug addicts the impact could be substantial and omitting these variables would be a major error.

The ease and cost of measurement must also be considered. It should be obvious that problems will exist in accurately measuring some criteria. For instance, there will be few individuals who will admit to committing crimes or other asocial behavior except after extensive (and costly) interviewing. The data collection costs may outweigh the value of the information. Yet, as illustrated, there are many criteria which are relatively easy to measure. There are others where, with a little thought, the development of new and less expensive operational measures could be accomplished. Unfortunately, however, too often experience has led potential impacts to be ignored, particularly for noneconomic impacts. In conclusion, it is our opinion that all potential impacts should be examined. Only where a strong and convincing case is made against an impact or criterion should it be omitted.

While the major emphasis in this section has been on measuring the impacts of health service programs, there is also the need to measure the impacts of

health training programs. These may include programs
directed toward educating health professionals in such
disciplines   as   medicine,   osteopathy,   dentistry,
optometry, podiatry, pharmacy, public health, health
services administration, and allied health.

Exercise 2-1

The President has given the Office of Management and Budget the authorization to consolidate a number of health and mental health programs into a single block grant to the states. Among the programs which are being considered for consolidation are family planning, migrant health, the community mental health and community health centers, and alcohol and drug treatment clinics.

You, as an analyst in the Office of Management and Budget, are asked to list the impacts of at least three of these programs. In making up the list you should attempt to demonstrate the degree of overlap between programs and their impacts.

Exercise 2-2

Provide detailed criteria to measure the impacts listed in Exercise 2-1.

Exercise 2-3

As an administrator of a family planning grantee agency at the state level, you are asked to outline the benefits expected to be derived from your clinics. You are to outline for the state's budget committee the basis on which you arrive at these estimates. To the extent possible, attempt to translate any perceived benefits into monetary values.

Exercise 2-4

In order to determine the impact of the Cedar City Community Health Center, the City Council has asked you as health planner to define the population affected by the health program. In the past, health officials have only considered clients who received health care treatment as having been impacted by the Center. Please discuss who else in Cedar City might be affected by the services provided by the Health Center, either directly or indirectly.

Suggested Readings

Bush, J., et al. "Cost-Effectiveness Using a Health Status Index: Analysis of the New York State PKU Screening Program," in Health Status Indexes: Proceedings of a Conference, R.L. Berg, ed. Chicago, Illinois: Hospital Research & Educational Trust, 1973.

Congress of the United States, Office of Technology Assessment. The Implications of Cost-Effectiveness Analysis of Medical Technology, Appendix D, "Values Ethics, and CBA in Health Care," August 1980.

Doherty, N., et al. "Cost Effectiveness Analysis and Alternative Health Care Progam for the Elderly," Health Services Research 12, Summer 1977.

Farshel, S., and Bush, J.W. "A Health Status Index and Its Application to Health Services Outcomes," Operations Research 18 (6), November-December 1970.

Klarman, H., et al. "Cost-Effectiveness Analysis Applied to the Treatment of Chronic Renal Disease," Medical Care 6, January-February 1968.

Murnaghn, J. "Health Indicators and Information Systems for the Year 2000," Annual Review of Public Health, 2, 1981.

Mushkin, S. "Knowledge and Choices in Health: Cost-Benefit Analysis in Health Policy Assessments," Washington, D.C., Georgetown University, Public Services Laboratory, 1977.

Veatch, R.M. "Justice and Valuing Lives," in Life Span, edited by R.M. Veatch, San Francisco, California: Harper and Row Publishing, 1979.

Weinstein, M. and Stason, W. Hypertension: A Policy Perspective, Cambridge, Massachusetts: Harvard University Press, 1976.

EVALUATION DESIGN

When evaluating health programs, we are trying to
determine their effects on clients, the government,
society, the health professional, and various other
parties. To do this we want to measure changes that
the program has created. As discussed in the last
chapter, we use changes in the health, social and
economic positions of individuals to measure the
influence of the program on society and the government. In order to determine the change which has
occurred with respect to an individual we need to know
what the person's health, experience, and situation
have been after a treatment episode or routine preventive care and what it would have been had there been
no health program or services offered.

Alternative Designs

This discussion centers around different designs which
may be used to measure the difference between the
actual experience of an individual once he or she
completed a health program and his or her expected
experience in the absence of the program.[19]
   The Case Study Design. Probably the simplest
design is the case study. Here, a new treatment
regimen or service is introduced to treat a particular
health problem, and the clients are observed after
receiving the intervention. Then, based on a guess as
to what would have happened to the clients had there
been no intervention, a judgment is made as to whether
or not the new method of treatment improved the lot of
the clients. This kind of design is quite common in

---

[19]In a primer such as this there are obvious limitations on our ability to cover the topic of experimental designs. We strongly urge the reader to
examine some of the theoretical literature dealing
with experimental design. We particularly recommend
Campbell and Stanley (33).

the evaluation of health programs. Many of the health programs begun in the 1960's grew out of experimental approaches to bring health services to the underserved. In many cases evaluation consisted of a description of the health program, or particular activities provided the underserved, e.g., early screening of children, innoculation campaigns, and more accessible emergency care.

There are a variety of major problems with the internal validity[20] of this design which can lead to overly positive conclusions about the program. First, there are events outside of the control of the evaluator which influence the observations that are made.[21] To give a concrete example, the success of substance abuse programs may depend largely on the environment to which the former addicts return rather than their in-program experiences. A heroin addict may not return to his or her habit if the street supply has dried up due to changes in enforcement or bad weather in the producing countries. Thus, there is a very great opportunity for the "post hoc ergo propter hoc" fallacy to exist. The evaluator implicitly says "In my opinion, the participant was better after the treatment; therefore, the treatment succeeded." Alternatively, a reformed alcoholic may have no intention of drinking but may give into the temptation as a result of stress caused by worsening national economic conditions which cause him or her to become unemployed. Here the program would be labelled a failure.

Second, the mere passage of time will influence the health status and the attitudes of most people.[22] This will be particularly true for the very young.

---

[20]Internal validity indicates that the design accurately measures the effects of the program on its participants.

[21]Campbell and Stanley (33) call this history.

[22]Campbell and Stanley (33) call this maturation.

For instance, teenagers may have very poor nutritional habits, which tend to improve as they become older. An evaluation of a nutrition education program which takes in teenagers, then, may find improved nutritional habits at age 21 which are due to changed attitudes about health rather than the program itself.

Another problem with the case study is that it is difficult to tell if there is a selection problem, particularly in the case of small-scale demonstration projects. There is the distinct possibility that such a project, an HMO for example, will be able to "cream"--take only the younger and healthier members of the community. It is not surprising, then, that over time, these HMO participants are found to do better in respect to health than the average person in the community.

Before-and-After Designs. While the case study approach has been used to make many actual policy decisions, health program evaluation has tended to follow a slightly more sophisticated design. The before-and-after design has been used in a number of government publications describing the benefits of health programs. The selection problem is removed since a comparison is being made with the same individuals. The other problems still remain, however. In fact, they become more serious for we are now considering a longer period of time in which events and maturation take place.

Probably the most serious problem in using observations before and after program participation for the evaluation of health and other social programs is the problem of "regression toward the mean." It is an observed phenomenon that in large populations which are examined over time those values at the extremes tend to move toward the middle. To give a specific example, if we look at the number of days sick for a cross section of the population, we find at one extreme individuals who have no illness during a year. At the other extreme are individuals who are sick for the entire year. If we make a cross-sectional analysis of sick days in the following year we find the same situation. Some individuals are well all the time, some individuals are totally incapacitated. If we follow the individuals in either of these categories, from one year to the next, however, we will find the individuals who are free from illness in the first year have a greater tendency to increase the number of days they are sick than does the population as a whole. This is not unreasonable for they have more days without illness to become sick. At the other extreme, the individuals who are sick for the entire first year will tend to have greater than average declines in days of sickness during the second year.

The problem in terms of the evaluation of health programs then is this: the individual who is eligible for treatment by these programs has serious health and social problems. Many alcoholics, for example, experience not only physical and mental disabilities, but are also unemployed, have family problems or are otherwise in severe need. These types of individuals are the ones who would be expected subsequently to have higher than average increases in their health, social and economic well-being because of regression toward the mean. When they therefore do show increases in these variables, it is difficult, if not impossible, to say what amount of the increase is due to the program and what amount is due to regression toward the mean.

We consequently have three major problems with simple before-and-after evaluations: the influence of extraneous events, the mere passage of time, and regression toward the mean.[23] An alternative formulation of before-and-after studies attempts to get around some of these problems. This method, labeled the interrupted time series, is to make repeated observations before the program or introduction of a new service and then repeated observations after the program. By the repeated observations some indication of the general trend caused by maturation should become evident. It should also show some of the

---

[23]There are other less important problems as well. See Campbell and Stanley (33).

regression toward the mean by evening out the cycle through which the individual is going if a number of observations over a considerable period of time can be made. However, this procedure may require continuing observations of the individuals over a long period before they are allowed to go into the program, which is obviously an expensive as well as time-consuming proposition and as such probably not practical in many instances.

Another alternative is to try to predict the expected before to after change through the use of multiple regression analysis. This procedure uses such independent variables as age to cover maturation, and growth in the economy to try to account for the problem of intervening events. The assumption is then made that the predicted experience of the individual resulting from the program are then net of these influences. This method, however, will not handle the regression toward the mean problem. Furthermore, it is very difficult to arrive at a regression model which accurately specifies the relationships of such variables as health status with explanatory variables.

Comparison Group[24] Designs. To get around a number of the problems involved in the before-and-after comparisons, evaluation of health programs may use a comparison group to represent the expected experience of the participants in the program in the absence of their participation. The key to the use of comparison groups lies in how well they represent the experience that program participants would have had in the absence of the program. If they do not closely

---

[24] We label as "comparison groups" any group whose expected characteristics and health outcomes would not be identical to those of the participants in the absence of program participation. A group which was randomly selected from the same population as the participants but not allowed to participate we label a "control group," since, if the numbers are large and the selection is truly random, they should be identical to the participants.

approximate the expected behavior and experience, all
of the problems previously discussed come into play.
Perhaps the easiest way to see this is to visualize a
program in nutritional health in which the participants are teenagers and the control group middle age
men and women. We can safely assume that the older
group will have more difficulty in changing life-long
eating habits than the teenagers who are still making
choices as to the types of food and drinking habits
they plan to follow. Therefore, particularly with a
before-and-after comparison, the program group (the
teenagers) would show greater gains that would the
comparison group of middle aged persons, regardless of
what the program did for the individuals involved.

Several sources may be used to secure members for
comparison groups.[25]   First, evaluations of on-going
programs have used individuals who had applied but who
did not enter the health program, e.g., an alcohol,
drug abuse, or health maintenance organization. This
is not a particularly good comparison group because
these individuals may differ from the program
participants in the following respects: (1) they did
not go into the program because they had alternative
means of care which they considered to offer better
prospects for success, (2) they did not go into the
program because they did not feel that they would be
able to follow the health regimens, (3) they were
excluded from the program because they did not meet

---

[25]The National Center for Health Statistics (NCHS) is
a primary source for selecting comparison group data
tapes. NCHS policy allows for the release of public
use data tapes when that can be done with existing
resources and in a manner which will not compromise
the confidentiality of respondents. Data from the
National Natality and Mortality Surveys, family
growth, health interview, national health and
nutrition examination surveys offer potentially rich
sources of data for the construct of such comparison
groups. See National Center for Health Statistics
(107).

the screening requirements, or (4) they lacked the motivation to enter the program. One could argue in the first case that the comparison group is superior to the program participants and in the other three cases that they are inferior (in terms of expected outcomes). A post-program observation of both groups should definitely expect to find some differences in their experiences, attitudes and behavior because of these four reasons. If a before-and-after design were used, it would be very difficult to say what interactions of differences between the groups and history, maturation and regression toward the mean would be expected--but they certainly could exist because of the selection process.

A similar type of situation exists for another common comparison group--one made up of individuals who applied to the program and who were deemed qualified but who did not enter. This comparison group is seemingly better than the one which includes persons who did not meet the entrance qualifications. It still may not be comparable, however, since the problems of self-selection (items 1, 2, and 4 above) or program selection (if the program took the most able of the qualified) remain.

Other studies have selected as comparison groups people in the same neighborhood who were in the same condition as the participants before the program. This group is one step removed from the clients in that they presumably did not apply for the program, because they lacked the motivation to do so. Questions arise as to what factors differentiate these individuals from those who entered the program and whether or not these factors would in turn lead to differences in the outcomes which are to be observed.

In all of these cases of comparison groups, one can attempt to match them with the client group through statistical control. To the extent that the two groups differ in identifiable characteristics which are thought to affect the outcome measures and which are quantifiable, the selection procedure or regression techniques can be used to take some account of these differences. Problems arises in that our models of what causes the outcomes are not well specified and they are measured with error so that the regression analyses will not measure all of the differences. Further, the matching process does not guarantee that the clients and comparison group members come from the same population. One person may be at the top of a low distribution and the other at the bottom of an overlapping, higher distribution. If this is the case they will regress to different means.

Also, there is a more basic problem in that we are unable to measure many of the variables which we believe affect the outcomes of health programs. For instance, motivation must be an important factor, but it is difficult to measure on a before-and-after basis--and impossible--on a retrospective basis. For these reasons, although they are desirable, statistical control methods are unlikely to solve the problems of the comparison group differences mentioned above.[26]

Random Control Groups. The answer to these problems is the random assignment of eligible persons to participate or to a control group. All of the persons who are qualified to enter the program must be contacted immediately before the start of the program to find out if they are still interested in entering. Those still wishing to be considered would then be split randomly with only one group assigned to actually enter the program. The second group would be given the regular services, if any, normally available to them. It is possible that this method could yield too small a number of persons included in the study who possess a particular characteristic which is important for analysis. If so, the group wishing to enter the program should be stratified by this characteristic. Then differing sampling proportions would be used from each of the strata. The sampling from each strata, however, would be random.

Random assignment procedures have the outstanding advantage of being statistically sound when they are

---

[26]For other approaches, see Cain (30) and Heckman (77).

applied to large groups. Known probabilities can be given to chance differences in the success of the two groups.[27] This would not be true of other means for selecting comparison gruops. Thus, any differences between the participants and control group observed in postprogram situations can be attributed to the program with known confidence levels.

Practical Problems of Random Assignment. Several problems are involved in the random selection of a control group. The first is the reluctance of health agencies to exclude fully qualified persons from receiving services. While such reluctance may be understandable, it appears shortsighted. Many health regimens, especially in the field of preventive health, are far from certain in relation to achieving positive effect. A mental health center, for example, may wish to test the effect of marriage seminars or stress management courses on the utilization of other health services during periods of marital crisis or separation. All clients are informed of the services, and a random sample of those showing interest are enrolled in the courses (or one of the two courses). The others receive no special treatment. It is only through measuring the utilization of health services by all groups that the center can know if the specially designed stress reduction courses actually effect utilization of other services.

It is true, however, that when using random assignment, decisions about which persons will enter a program may be different than those which would have been made in the absence of the evaluation. While this might not greatly concern the evaluator, it doubtlessly will be of great importance to the operating staff of the programs which are being evaluated. They may view the random selection procedure as basically denying the professional criteria which they use for program admission. As such they may believe

―――――――――――――――――

[27]For instance we can say that 95 times out of 100 a difference as large as we observe is not due to chance.

that the evaluation is harmful to the program and the clients. To service providers random assignment is effectively denying services to persons who have sought them in the belief that such services would improve their health. Furthermore, it is only natural that the program staff who must be held accountable for the program and their own work should believe that it does help the participants. (It would be a sorry situation if health care providers did not believe that they and their programs were accomplishing good.) The major critique of random assignment boils down to the question: "When one realizes that health programs have been established primarily to assist individuals to better their situation rather than for research purposes, how can one deny them services that they need and have requested? Moreover, how can they continue to be denied service over a period of time despite their urgent need and interest?"

There are several possible answers to this question. First, and probably the most important, is the question--"How can you be sure that the health program in question actually does assist the participants to better their health?" (This is especially true of experimental health, alcohol and drug treatment programs.) Many new health programs have come into being and grown very quickly in the last several years; e.g., genetic counseling services, adolescent pregnancy programs, and marriage counseling programs. Yet, they have been subjected to constant revision. These changes presumably occurred because the programs were either not operating to the benefit of the participants or they could be improved considerably. We have seen major changes in the emphasis of many health programs in recent years. For example, many programs now give much greater attention to patient education and self care than was formerly provided. The nature of health planning also changed rather significantly with the passage of the Health Planning and Resources Development Act of 1974. Mental health treatment now emphasizes community-based care rather than institutional care. The recent infusion of the hospice concept for the care of terminally ill patients is another of the many examples of significant change that could be cited. Presumably all of these changes occurred because it was believed that individuals served by earlier programs could be better served by other programs or no programs at all. These changes did not come about, however, until literally hundreds of thousands of individuals had participated. Typically there was a delay of several years between the inception of a program and the gathering of data to show that it was not producing the most desirable outcomes. These individuals did not receive the services which were subsequently determined to have been more appropriate for them, and they even could have been harmed by the services that they did receive.[28] What we have here is a situation somewhat similar to the doctor who presents a quack "miracle cure" for cancer to his patients: (1) some seem to benefit from it; (2) others survive it; (3) some, because they have taken the "cure", do not seek any other means of treatment and subsequently are worse off; and (4) finally, others die from the treatment itself. One need only postulate the third alternative to see the risks that are inherent in health programs not being properly evaluated.

On strictly practical grounds there are often not enough openings in many health program services to satisfy the universe of need. Almost always there is a rationing of program services. Ideally, the services will be assigned to those most needing them. Usually, however, assignment is on the basis of some other, less beneficial criterion, such as on a first come, first served basis for those who qualify for the program or those most likely to pay for the services. The random assignment technique will not reduce the amount of services provided or the

---

[28]One could argue that many of the individuals who went through programs were harmed by them. The individuals who were confined in mental institutions without receiving treatment would be a good example, or clients heavily exposed to x-rays or unnecessary drug therapy.

the eligibility of the clients. It will merely change which qualified people receive the services, and may more equitably distribute the benefits of the program by giving qualified individuals an equal chance to participate.

Another problem with the random assignment technique is that it requires more extensive selection than would normally occur. Under ordinary conditions it is only necessary to interview, test, and refer persons to the program until all openings are filled. With random assignment enough additional persons must be found who also qualify for the program so that a control group of adequate size can be selected. Since the services selected for evaluation will form only a very small part of each program, the increase in cost will be relatively small. It should be viewed as a cost of the research which will be well repaid in terms of the accuracy of the results.

Since the control group will not receive any treatment it may have a higher rate of attrition in terms of gathering follow-up information. If particular segments of the control group are omitted when outcomes are measured, this may introduce bias. To counter the problem of attrition, researchers can provide special vigilance to the control group by collecting alternate addresses, tracking addresses carefully, and planning for increased time and effort to service this population. Staff may also collect as much information at the initial screening on client characteristics that are relevant both to possible attrition rates and the treatment process. Researchers who are unable to offer money incentives to control group members may compensate participants by assurances of test results, offers of medical, psychological, or other services to enhance their participation over time.[29]   If the control group and

---

[29]Guerney (73), for example, recruited members for a demonstration therapy program telling them that they had a 1/3 chance of not being selected for treatment. He told them they would, nevertheless, be paid

the experimental group are identified at the start of
a project, efforts can be made to keep track of
persons in them. This will improve the response rate
for the evaluation and reduce the costs of follow-
up. The choice of retrospective comparison groups
usually involves trying to contact persons with whom
there has been no link for many months. Many cannot
be located, and a great deal of time and effort is
spent trying to locate the others. Thus, the use of
the random assignment technique may lead to a lower
total cost for the evaluation. Finally, while the
random assignment technique requires a longer time
period from the start to the end of the evaluation
than would a retrospective study, for a new program or
a changing program the two techniques will yield their
findings at the same time.[30]

Theoretical Problems with Random Assignment.
Unfortunately, while the randomized assignment design
insures an accurate assessment of programs for individuals who have enrolled in them, like all other
designs there can be a variety of external validity
problems (i.e., there are problems in generalizing
beyond the particular group which has been studied).
These same problems apply to the nonrandom designs
discussed earlier. They include the following.
(1) The pretest observation and the treatment itself
may interact. For instance, if before a preventive
dentistry program I am asked about my sugar consumption, I may well concentrate on reducing sugar intake
when I get into the program. Thus the fact that the
pretest observation has been made may influence my
subsequent behavior in the experiment. (2) Another
similar problem, which Campbell and Stanley (33) call
"reactive arrangements" and which is more generally
known as the "Hawthorne effect," is probably more

$10.00 for testing on measures at two different points
in time.

[30]The reader interested in further arguments for and
against random assignment should see Boruch (19) and
Campbell and Boruch (32).

important and more difficult to handle. This occurs
when the individuals realize that they are receiving
special treatment and so perform differently simply
because they are participating in an experiment.
Similarly, and possibly more important for health
programs, the providers of services (the staff) knowing that they are being evaluated may perform
differently than they do normally. (3) The selection
of the groups to be studied may be such that they are
not truly typical of the general population. For
instance, a small pilot program, simply because it is
small, may be more selective in choosing clients than
a national program might be. A more serious problem
is often a tendency to generalize findings to other
groups beyond those which have been studied. For
instance, most health programs are voluntary, and
through an experimental design accurate measurement of
the program's effects for participants can be made.
These measurements, however, may not apply to the same
program when participation is made compulsory as would
be the case for court ordered participation in a
mental health program. (4) Accurate assessments may
be given a certain history of events, but these may
not hold for other conditions. For example, it is
possible to measure accurately the effects of a program that provides outpatient mental health services
in a period of economic prosperity--which will not be
an accurate measurement for a period of decline since
estimates of self-worth are based somewhat on economic
success. (5) In a somewhat similar vein, there is the
criticism that evaluations often examine as a single
entity a health program which consists of a number of
different services. These services need not be
consistent from one location to the next. Conceivably, we can have a situation where a program
worked in one city because of a charismatic director,
but it may not be possible to recreate that charisma
in leaders in a number of other cities. Consequently
the program may not be as successful there. Yet, the
evaluations do not examine the components of the
program and the reasons for its success io failure.
The program is treated as a "black box" that is not
opened to examine the contents. (6) Finally, it is

difficult to maintain randomized designs for long
periods of time, once they are implemented.

These problems can be handled in a variety of
ways. The pretest interacting with the treatment is
probably the easiest to handle. One need only exclude
the pretest. The use of the "post test only design"
may also help remove any Hawthorne effect for the
participants, since they will not know they are being
evaluated. In terms of the program staff one can try
not to notify them than an evaluation is taking
place. Of course, this is usually difficult to do.
Alternatively, one can evaluate a sufficiently large
group of projects over a long enough period so that
only a small proportion of any given program is to be
sampled. This makes it extremely difficult for the
program staff to decide who gets special treatment.
For the problem of self-selection and creaming one can
attempt to diversify the types of program participants
to be studied.[31] One can repeatedly evaluate so that
the program is studied under many different conditions
to account for the problem of generalizing beyond one
set of economic conditions. If there is a "black box"
problem, one can attempt to observe the operation of
the program or to disassemble the program into its
components and then evaluate the effectiveness of each
of these.

Another possible problem with random assignment
comes about because nonselection for a health program
can conceivably have a negative effect on outcomes for
the control group. If services are refused and the
individual is told that he or she is ineligible for
the program, this may be one more of a set of disap-
pointments which reduce desire, motivation, and
ability to function. If this is the case, then the
selection process itself must be considered as exter-
nally invalidating the results by giving a positive

---

[31]If the criteria for self-selection and creaming are
known then these can be included either directly or
with an instrumental variable in the model. Such
criteria are seldom known, however.

bias to the measured success of the program. Therefore, one must devise some kind of assignment process
that is neutral in its effect on those who are to
serve as the control group. Unfortunately, it is very
difficult to design a placebo health services program. Since many health programs are widely touted in
the press and in various outreach functions, it is
difficult to tell individuals that they do not really
want to enter the program because we are not sure it
would be good for them. Whereas some health programs
may not produce drastic changes in health status or
behavior for an individual, it is hard to design one
which will have no positive or negative effects and
yet not be viewed as a sham by the participants. This
problem is a major issue which is as yet unresolved in
program evaluation. The answer probably lies in
honesty. The potential clients should be told that
some will not be enrolled and that the decision will
be made randomly.

Finally we come to the problem of lack of independence between the treatment group and the control
group. For example, a program may be designed to
provide preventive medical services in a small community where there is only a single physician. In the
absence of the program those receiving care might be
distributed randomly among the population; when the
program does exist all health care is provided to
program clients and none is provided to the control
group. In this situation the control group is not a
good proxy for the experience of the program clients
in the absence of the program. As postulated, in the
absence of the program there would be random distribution of the care, and some of the persons who subsequently participated in the program would have received care. With the program, however, no one in the
control group will receive care. In this case there
would be an overstatement of the incremental benefits
of the program.

The lack of independence may also work in the
opposite direction if the benefits of program participation are transferred from the clients to the control
group. Such a situation is most likely to occur when
there is close contact between the clients and control

group members. This may occur when they all come from
a small area and when the program provides information
which is easy to convey, such as nutritional information   or   information   relating   to   exercise   or
pregnancy. In these circumstances there is an under-
statement of program benefits because some of the
benefits of the program will accrue to the control
group. The purpose of the control group is to show
what would have happened in the absence of any program
and if the control group is influenced in any way by
the existence of the program, it does not truly
reflect the experience of the participants if there
were no program.

These problems are not easy to resolve. One alternative is to conduct the evaluation while the program
is still small, relative to the population of a given
community. (If the evaluated program is providing
preventive health care to one hundred persons in New
York City, its impact on the health of people in the
city as a whole will be extremely small.) The evaluator, however, should be aware of the threat to
external validity due to the lack of independence of
the experimental and control groups, and should
attempt to prevent the participants from becoming such
a large fraction of the total so that they overshadow
the control group.

Alternatives to Random Assignment. In the situation where random assignment is not allowed because it
is believed to interfere with the enforcement of
strict eligibility requirements an alternative is the
regression-discontinuity design. Program managers are
asked to specify all selection criteria that they wish
to use and then to rank all applicants by these
criteria. They then follow these rankings in selecting individuals for admission.[32] For instance, all
individuals with incomes below $3,000 may be admitted,

---

[32]Exceptions who are admitted although they do not
meet the criteria and persons excluded even though
they meet the criteria are identified and not
considered in the evaluation.

and all those above excluded, or all persons exhibit-
ing certain characteristics on a medical screening
inventory may be entered and those without the characteristics excluded. The postprogram outcomes are then
regressed separately on the rankings of the two groups
(e.g., incomes or characteristics). If significant
differences between the two groups appear at the cut-
off point ($3,000 or a certain set of characteristics)
this would indicate that the program had an impact, at
least at that point.

  There are several obvious virtues to this
procedure. It allows the program managers freedom to
make all program assignments, it does not involve any
unusual effort on their part, and it can be adopted to
many types of programs. However it also has some
shortcomings. First, there should be no natural
discontinuities in the outcome measures. Second, the
effect of the program is only measured at one point--
the technique does not allow a determination of
whether the program would be equally effective for
persons with incomes of $10,000 or different health
problems. Third, if the relationship between the
selection variable and the dependent variable is not
properly defined (e.g., a linear regression is used
when the data are not linear), incorrect estimates may
occur. Finally the technique does not solve any of
the external validity problems discussed earlier.[33]

  Another alternative is often proposed if the
evaluation seeks only to determine which of several
programs is preferable. Persons qualified and
interested in participating would be randomly assigned
to one of the programs. Recruitment would not exceed

---

[33]The reader is strongly urged to read Campbell (31)
and Boruch and Riecken (20), pp. 87-116 for more
discussion of the regression-discontinuity design.
For instance, it might be argued that if the
relationships on both sides of the discontinuity are
properly described and identical, then one can
estimate the impact of the program at points other
than the discontinuity.

the number of program openings and a control group
whose members do not enter any of the programs would
not be necessary. Persons in each program would serve
as control group members for comparison with the
clients of other programs.

Notwithstanding the advantages of this type of
analysis, there is a problem in that it gives the
increments in the benefits of one program over another
as opposed to the increment in the cost. This does
not yield what it is really necessary to know: some
measure of the ratios of the total benefits to the
total costs for the two programs. Only in the situation where we know the cost and benefits of one program as opposed to no program or in that situation
where the two programs have highly comparable costs
can accurate interprogram comparison be made.

The Choice of an Experimental Group

Of the persons eligible to enroll in a health program,
some will cancel appointments or drop out before they
enter, others will enter the program but will leave
before they complete treatment, and finally, others
will complete the full program. None of the control
or comparison group members will participate in the
program. Some studies have argued that only those
individuals who participated in all required program
services or only those people who completed the program and properly followed after care protocols should
be included in the calculation of the program's
benefits. Such a procedure must make two assumptions
to be correct: (1) the individuals who did not go into
the program and the individuals who dropped out of the
program were totally unaffected by it, and (2) these
individuals did not differ in their expected post-
program experience from the clients who completed the
program. Such assumptions probably are not warranted.

It is quite obvious that those individuals who
dropped out of the program (e.g., a preventive
dentistry program) gained some knowledge or health
regimens while they participated which might
subsequently impact on their health. On the other
hand, they may have lost time searching for a job, and

missed other types of opportunities while engaged in program activities. There may also be a stigma attached in that employers might consider the dropouts unstable because they did not complete the program. The individuals who did not enter the program or who dropped out of it also may feel rejection or lowered personal self-worth. Lowered self esteem could subsequently affect their functioning in many aspects of their lives. Similarly, the program may affect all the people who complete it, not only those who make use of it. Beneficial or negative changes in their health status may occur among program participants even if they do not appear to be affected. Consequently, the effects of the program on all participants must be examined if a full accounting is to be achieved.[34]

With regard to the second assumption, the control group is used to represent the aggregate experience of all persons who were selected for the program. Unless the clients are a homogenous group, which earlier we argued was unlikely, it will be necessary to separate the control group into segments corresponding to those who receive full services and of those receiving only partial treatment in order to make comparisons. Such a division will be very difficult since identification of the factors which lead individual clients to receive services will be required. As discussed previously, our ability to measure and model such factors is very limited. For instance, a preventive dental program may show fewer cavities for persons who remained in the program longer. Yet, we will probably never know if extended participation or greater motivation is the primary causal agent.

---

[34]This does not mean that no distinctions should be made between different types of program participants. The analysis should seek to determine the differences which exist between completers and dropouts in order to determine the necessity of reducing the proportion of dropouts or the possibility of altering the program activities.

Measuring Degree of Treatment

Differential treatment intervention is always a problem for the experimental group. Counseling sessions for participants in a drug treatment program, for example, may vary from a few hours to many hours or weeks of group and individual sessions. Sometimes the members never receive any of the services. The experiences of some experimental group members may, therefore, resemble the control group members more closely than the experiences of other experimental group members. It is particularly important, therefore, to collect information on the type and amount of services received in order to account for such variation and to compare participants who received frequent and intensive treatment with those receiving relatively small and infrequent amounts of treatment.[35]

The Timing of Impact Measurement

Since a major purpose of evaluation is to affect policy relating to the program's operation, there are a variety of pressures which move toward early measurement of the impacts and costs of the program. Policymakers and politicans, anxious for pilot programs which appear useful for expansion to a nationwide status, often do not want to wait for the results of the evaluation before proceeding. Health administrators want to know which of the alternative funding possibilities are most effective so that they can make their annual allocations. Program managers want results which will justify their program to policy makers and the public and which will permit them to alter their program to make it operate more efficiently.

Yet, pilot programs need time so administrators can work out the "kinks" in their operations. The programs' administrators must: 1) establish a series of procedures for treating clients; 2) hire and train

---

[35]See Fitzgerald, Hormuth and Cook (66).

staff, weeding out those staff members who cannot perform; 3) publicize the program and attract suitable clients; and 4) operationalize the program. Undoubtedly, these steps will require time before the program can operate efficiently. If the program is evaluated before this has happened, there will probably be a downward bias in the estimate of the program's impact.[36] In addition, it is necessary for sufficient time to pass after the program treatment for the transitory effects of the program to be dissipated. Finally, seasonal factors should be removed from the data by allowing at least a full year to pass after treatment before impact measurement.[37]

For these reasons it makes sense to delay the evaluation of programs until they have operated for at least six months. Then measurements of program impact should occur one year after the client has concluded treatment of some kind (although earlier measurements are not precluded). Evaluations should also be made at three or five year intervals after the program clients have first enrolled to find the longer run impacts. In all cases care should be taken to insure that the data are collected for identical time periods for both the experimental and control groups. Otherwise, problems with cyclical fluctuations may arise. Variables such as number of days sick and total earnings should be measured for the entire postprogram period as well as for the individual years. Such measurements will demonstrate the total effect of the program and changes in program interventions over time.

---

[36]There can be an upward bias, however, if the program "creams" its clients at the beginning.

[37]This is seen by using an outpatient mental health treatment program as an example. If the measurement is made on attitudes during a three-month period ending in September, considerably different results may be obtained than if the measurement is made for three months ending in March.

The Choice of Retrospective or Concurrent Data Collection

One can identify clients and comparison group members who participated in the health program at some earlier period and gather information retrospectively relative to their treatment. Alternatively, data collection can occur by identifying a group of future program participants and control or comparison group members and then gathering information from or about them over succeeding periods. There are merits to both procedures.

Retrospective studies provide results faster; they do not require waiting for the postprogram period to occur before measurements are made. This shorter elapsed time from the decision to conduct the evaluation to the presentation of its findings is the reason most evaluations have been conducted in this manner. Another argument in its favor is that there will be no "Hawthorne effect" since the individuals and staff do not know that data will subsequently be gathered about them. Further, retrospective data gathering does not require that the evaluation be built directly into the program's operation. This makes advance planning unnecessary.

Offsetting these factors, concurrent data collection offers several important benefits. First, it is impossible to have control groups in a retrospective study because random assignment is impossible after the program has ended. It should also be noted that it will be difficult to implement the regression discontinuity design on a retrospective basis as the selection criteria will usually not be made explicit in normal program operations. Therefore, retrospective studies must construct ad hoc comparison groups from whatever records that may exist. This will usually involve substantial difficulties since programs seldom maintain information on nonclients and to the extent that these lists are incomplete or inaccurate, biases may be introduced. Next, data gathered on a retrospective basis are much more likely to involve response errors. The longer the period to be covered, the more likely will be memory lapses. Also, studies show that accurate attitudinal measures are very difficult to collect on a retrospective basis because perceptions of past attitudes are altered by intervening events. Finally, as argued earlier, retrospective studies are more likely to have inadequate response rates. It is more difficult and costly to try to locate individuals after contact has been severed than to maintain contact with individuals currently under treatment.

We find the set of arguments for concurrent studies to be much the stronger. In our opinion the opportunity to use a control group or the regression discontinuity design outweighs the time consideration. We believe that valid data are much better than early, but inaccurate information. Also the greater ease and lower cost of concurrent data collection have much appeal. Therefore, we strongly urge its use.

Collecting Data on the Impacts

Direct contact has been the basic method used to collect information about the program clients and control group members. Special studies have usually used personal interviews, while the typical program follow-up system has relied primarily on mail questionnaires and telephone interviews. The problems with direct contact are well known: besides being time consuming and costly, response rates on personal interviews seldom are above 90 percent and those on mail and telephone surveys are considerably lower.[38] Yet, for many variables which are affected by health programs direct contact may be the only source of information.

The random selection technique presented earlier should reduce some of the problems associated with contacting individuals. Since the individuals for whom data will subsequently be collected are known from the

---

[38]For an excellent review of these issues we suggest that reader see Weiss (153).

start of the program, special efforts can be made to remain in contact with them during and after the program. For instance, sample members may be given stamped cards to report all changes of address, the names of relatives and others who would know the location of the respondent could be secured, and the need for follow-up information could be impressed on the sample members. This should aid in achieving a higher response rate and reducing the costs of the survey, particularly when contact needs to be maintained for a period of at least one year after the program.

Because of the variety of information on dependent variables needed at the end of the first year following the program, personal contact appears to be the best technique to use for the first evaluation of a health program. Subsequent evaluations may consider the use of existing records.[39]

Sample Size

The problem of how many clients or comparison group members should be examined is always a very difficult one. The usual rule of thumb is to include as many as the budget will allow. At times more sophisticated justifications must be provided. In these situations the best strategy is to contact a sampling expert. If one is not available, the simplest calculation is dependent on the disperson of the variable being studied and the level of precision desired. The formula for the standard error of the difference between means for the participants and control or comparison group members is:

---

[39]A problem becoming increasingly more important is the reluctance of various government agencies subject to federal and state "privacy acts" to provide data for identifiable individuals. Without the ability to link records for individuals many of the economies associated with the use of existing data sets are lost.

$$\bar{Sx} = \sigma/ \ N(\pi)(1 - \pi)$$

where: is the standard deviation of the variable, N
the sample size, π the proportion of the sample in the
program, and $1 - \pi$ the proportion in the control or
comparison group. To solve for N,

$$N = \frac{(\sigma/\bar{Sx})^2}{(\pi)(1 - \pi)}$$

Thus, a larger sample size will be needed as: 1) the
disperson of the dependent variable (σ) increases the
confidence interval, 2) the precision $(\sigma/Sx)^2$ desired
increases, and 3) the proportion of participants in
the sample (π) moves away from fifty percent.

Sources of Data on Comparison Group Members

When retrospective studies are made and require the
use of existing records to identify persons to serve
as members of comparison groups, the evaluator may
turn to several sources of data. If he or she desires
to identify individuals who applied for a health
program but who did not begin treatment (probably the
preferred comparison group for retrospective studies),
the evaluator must rely on records which usually are
found, if they exist, in the local offices of the
project or grantee agency. The use of such records
requires the identification of the facilities to be
studied, the contacting of the local administrators, a
detailed search of their records to ensure a complete
list, and the selection of a sample from this list.
Since these records probably will not contain any
information about the individuals after the completion
of the program, the individuals will have to be contacted to make certain that none of the comparison
group subsequently participated in the program. These
procedures will be both costly and time consuming.
Alternatively, comparison groups may be constructed
from among individuals similar to clients who have
been surveyed in other studies.

The Choice of Variables for Analysis

To conduct an evaluation of a health program, it is necessary to measure the relationships between the program impacts (the dependent variables) and a variety of independent variables, including the personal characteristics of clients, the program services, the interventions and the conditions under which the health program operates.

Personal Independent Variables. These independent variables are particularly relevant for comparing program clients with the members of the control or comparison group to discover whether differences exist between the groups which may affect the program impacts. It is necessary to include in the analysis as many variables as possible which are correlated with both program participation and the dependent variables. However most relevant dependent variables with which evaluations of health programs deal are functions of more than one independent variable. To omit some variables in the analysis may lead to distorted conclusions due to correlation or interaction among these variables and those independent variables which are included in the analysis. The analyses should treat all of the independent variables simultaneously.

The use of simple cross tabulations to isolate such relationships will be inadequate in most cases. For instance, the effects of race, age, occupation and place of residence on health status are all interrelated.[40] Yet each of these effects should be

---

[40]Among the items recommended for a minimum patient data set at hospital discharge includes: personal identification, date of birth, sex, race and ethnicity, residence, hospital certification, admission and discharge data, physician identification, diagnoses, procedures and dates, dispostion of patient, and expected principal source of payment. See U.S. Department of Health and Human Services (143).

distinguished. To cross tabulate by all of these variables would involve so many cells that the sample would have to be enormous. In addition, the tables would be so large as to be unmanageable. Therefore, multivariate techniques should be used in the evaluations to discover and test the statistical significance of any relationships which are observed. Multiple regression and correlation techniques can be performed with a much smaller sample than cross tabulations and permit easy interpretation of the findings.

Evaluations should examine the effects of the programs on groups of clients for other reasons too. The analyses should determine whether or not a particular program will benefit certain target groups for whom the program was designed, as well as find which interventions serve the groups best. For most health programs, independent variables should be included in the analysis to represent different groups with high percentages among the sick or disabled, as well as other groups traditionally underserved, e.g., blacks, Mexican-Americans, Native Americans, the aged, and persons in high risk occupations. The degree of success should be measured for such characteristics of the program participants as age, sex, race, ethnic group, number of dependents, family size, education, diagnosis, etc. Many personal characteristics are listed in Table 3-1.

It is also necessary to treat personal characteristics in the evaluation in order to improve the efficiency of the programs. Programs will have varying results for different types of people. The personal variables in Table 3-1 can also be used to determine which individuals receive the greatest benefits from each intervention, and individuals can be assigned so that the success of each program is maximized. The attitudinal variables in Table 3-1 may be particularly useful for these purposes.

This assignment process may be in conflict with the desire to benefit certain target groups, however, because these groups receive lower benefits than do other persons from all of the program's interventions. In this case, knowledge of which interventions

Table 3-1

Personal Variables Affecting Health Program Success

Characteristics

access to transportation
age
attitudes of other family members toward health care
   and prevention
dietary and nutritional practices
educational level
eligibility for different types of income maintenance
   and health insurance support
employment status at enrollment
family composition including:
      age and sex of other family members
      number of dependents
      number of other family members
family income and health of other family members
health and disability history
intelligence level
level of alcohol, drug, and tobacco use
licenses and certificates
marital status
mental health history
military service
occupation and salary level
previous program participation and utilization of
   health services
prior mobility
race and ethnic background
sex
skills and abilities
socioeconomic background

Attitudes

attitude toward safety, driving practices
attitude toward health and mental health
degree of independence

Table 3-1 continued

Attitudes

general disposition
level of maturity
motivation to engage in preventive health program
perceived limitations on ability to curtail drinking
  and smoking
self-confidence
self-esteem
willingness to change dietary practice

serve which groups best will be useful, nevertheless, because it still will be more efficient to allocate the target groups to those program services where they receive the largest benefits. If there are still program openings, the individuals who would have the greatest expected benefits would be encouraged to enroll.

Program Component Independent Variables. Most health programs consist of a set of activities and services, and many of these are common to several groups, e.g., a drug treatment program may provide ten hours group counseling, twenty hours supervised work, five hours individual therapy a week. It would be extremely useful in modifying existing programs and in the planning of new programs to know which of the activities are most effective for various types of participants. It would also be desirable to have information on the best combinations of interventions or components. To the extent that the length and nature of the intervention supplied to individuals differ within or between health programs, multivariate techniques can be used to identify effective interventions. If evaluations examine programs which include a variety of interventions and where the length of the interventions vary they should include as independent variables the amount of each service performed in a program (this will usually be expressed in terms of hours spent per participant) and, if possible, a measure of quality. Evaluations should also examine the type and qualifications of the health professionals who provide health services. In this way individual staff characteristics may be examined as a factor effecting health program outcomes. Greater clarification may also be given as to the proper use of para-professionals and other support staff in the provision of services.

Exogenous Independent Variables. Health programs will also differ in their effectiveness depending on the characteristics of the location and the circumstances in which they operate. Possible factors affecting program success are nearly limitless and depend on the nature of the program under discussion. A partial list of potential factors includes:

climate, air quality, the social and cultural norms of the population relative to life styles, e.g., drinking, eating, drug and tobacco use. These factors should be included in the analysis as independent variables to determine under what conditions the programs are most effective and which programs (and interventions) are most effective under particular conditions.

Determining Proper Program Size--Measuring at the Margin

A basic question which the evaluation should answer is, "What should be the health program's size?" (including the possibility that the answer may be that no health program is justified for a particular community). Ideally, the evaluation would provide an accounting of the total benefits derived from the program at each possible level of program activity. The decision maker could then compare various health programs and allocate expenditures to yield the level of activity for each which would maximize the total return on the total expenditure. To do this, resources would be allocated so that each additional dollar was spent on the program which yielded the greatest return for that dollar, given the distribution of previous expenditures.

To date, however, evaluations of health programs have not presented these data. Rather, average benefits have been calculated for a program at fixed levels of program activity. In order to make program size decisions, users of these analyses have had to assume that the average benefits of different programs have a direct relationship to the benefits at the margin, i.e., that adding a person to a program with a high average benefit will be more beneficial than enrolling the person in a program with a lower average benefit. Only if this assumption is true, however, will the decision maker end up with the optimal allocation of his or her resources.

There are techniques which can be used to roughly approximate the effects of changes in program size. One technique is to relate the absolute and relative sizes of the program in different locations to the level of program success in those areas. There will be a wide range of program sizes which may be used to predict the effects of program growth or cutbacks. For example, if a health program has higher average benefits in areas where only five percent of the underserved participate as compared with areas with higher participation rates, program expansion to include more underserved people would be expected to reduce average benefits, all other factors held constant.

As changes occur in program size, this will usually mean changes in the type of program clients. For instance, small programs may "cream" and only recruit relatively low risk clients, while larger programs will have to dig deeper and enroll people who may benefit less directly from a program, e.g., a pregnancy prevention program expands to include those teenagers who are sexually active as well as those already pregnant, or those who have had no former pregnancy. It is likely that programs have differential effects depending on the type of participants. Therefore, if the evaluations can determine the average effects of the programs on different groups of clients this can be used to predict the effects of changes in program size with increased participation by particular groups.[41]   Similarly, if changes in program size involve changes in program services, knowledge of the average benefits for each service or intervention will be useful. As the number of evaluations increase, more exact measures of the effects of program size will gradually become available.

---

[41]The average benefits of a group may not equal the benefits for the last member of that group who participates in the program. If, however, the effects of the programs on the groups under consideration differ greatly, the use of average benefits for subgroups will probably approximate more closely the marginal effects of the change in program size than will the average return for all program participants.

Presumably the experience of older programs and program activities can then be transferred to new ones.
Meanwhile, however, we should seek to measure the
impact of programs on subgroups of the clients, for
particular services of the program, and in different
areas.

Exercise 3-1

Horizon Health Center (HHC), which serves Horizon
City but not its suburbs, is eager to expand its
services to the community. One of the areas it has
identified as needing attention is preventive health
care. A course has begun at HHC focussing on diet,
exercise, body chemistry and self administered physical examination. The first class attending the course
was enthusiastic about it, and the course was favor-
ably reported in the local newspaper. In that news
story, the president of HHC was quoted as saying, "It
is our duty to serve all of the people of Horizon. We
will provide this course to any resident of Horizon
City who wishes to enroll. Furthermore, no one will
have to wait to enroll. We will run as many sections
of the course as are necessary to accommodate all
potential students."

Dr. M.A. Lee, the Director of the State Health
Education Department, reading the news story, questions if this course should be offered at other health
clinics in the state. She asks you to evaluate the
success of the course as it has operated at HHC.
Before you actually begin the study you are required
to present her with an outline which: (1) shows the
research design you will use to measure the changes
caused by the course, (2) present alternative designs,
and (3) present arguments for your suggested design
against the alternatives. Prepare such an outline.

Exercise 3-2

The Horizon Institute for Advanced Design has been
contracted to evaluate the impact of the mental health
services provided at the Cedar City Mental Health
Center Program. The Mental Health Center has a month-
ly intake of over 200 clients, with a waiting list of
approximately 50 clients at any one time. Since there
are many more people in need of services than the
Center is able to provide, many prospective clients
must be referred to other private and public social
service agencies after an initial administrative
intake. Basically the Center administrator wants to

know:

1. If the Center is serving clients who are best able
    to profit from the program provided at Cedar City
    Center.

2. If the level of functioning of clients improves
    significantly as compared to prior levels of
    functioning, or other clients referred elsewhere.

3. If services must be reduced with proposed funding
    cutbacks, where should they be curtailed.

The Horizon Institute has available all Center
records for the past three years, and has been allowed
a 12-month period for collecting additional data.
Please outline a design which would enable the Center
administrator to make such decisions and also defend
his or her program before county and state management.

Suggested Readings

Campbell, D.T. and Boruch, R.F.   "Making the Case for
Randomized Assignment to Treatments by Considering the
Alternatives: Six Ways in Which Quasi-Experimental
Evaluations in Compensatory Education Tend to Under-
estimate Effect," Evaluation and Experiment: Some
Critical Issues in Assessing Social Programs, C.A.
Bennett and A.A. Lumsdaine, eds., New York: Academic
Press, 1975.

Campbell, D.T. and Stanley, J.C.   Experimental and
Quasi-Experimental Designs for Research, Chicago:
Rand McNally and Company, 1971.

Cook, T.D. and Campbell, D.T.   Quasi-Experimentation
Design and Analysis Issues for Field Settings, New
York: Rand McNally, 1979.

Cook, T.D. and Reichardts, C.S., eds.   Qualitative and
Quantitative Methods in Evaluation Research, Beverly
Hills: Sage Publications, 1979.

Fitzgerald, N.M., Hormuth, S.E. and Cook, T.D.
"Quasi-Experimental Methods in Community Psychology
Research," in E.C. Susskind and D.C. Klein, eds.,
Knowledge Building in Community Psychology, New
York: Holt, Reinhart, and Winston, 1981.

Stahler, G. and Tash, W.R. eds.   Innovative Approaches
in Mental Health Program Evaluation, New York:
Academic Press, 1982.

Wholey, J.S., et al.   Federal Evaluation Policy:
Analyzing the Effects of Public Programs, Washington,
D.C.:   The Urban Institute, 1970.

THE COSTS OF HEALTH PROGRAMS

No program provides its benefits free; something must be given up in order to derive them. Resources which are devoted to health programs cannot be used to produce other goods and services. For instance, society by devoting human resources to conduct maternal and child health programs loses the services of the medical staff for alternative assignments in or outside the health field. Thus, the costs of health programs should be considered to be their opportunity costs--the value of the alternative benefits which are foregone because of the programs' presence.

Estimating Opportunity Costs

It is usually impossible, however, to identify what benefits are foregone and to place a value on them, especially for comprehensive health programs. For instance, what production would be lost if society chose to institute a national health insurance plan? What potential output did society give up by providing medical services to the poor and elderly under Medicaid and Medicare? Consequently, because of the measurement problems, the opportunity cost is often assumed to equal (or at least be proportionate to) the market price of the resources which go into the program. This assumption rests on competitive market theory which states that in a perfectly competitive market, each marginal factor of production will be paid an amount equal to the value of its product in its present and next best alternative use. Thus, in perfect competition the amount paid for producing a product will reflect the value of the opportunities foregone. (This means that registered nurses in a maternal and child health program will be paid an amount equal to the value of their output in their next best occupation, say, as instructors in a local college.)
There are many problems with the application of this theory. Health programs do not usually operate in situations of perfect competition. Most health

programs involve the government purchasing resources which do not have large, well-defined competitive markets with many alternative buyers. For example, the number of purchasers of acute care hospital buildings and personnel is quite limited. In most geographic areas, there are usually only a few hospitals. In addition, the government is not a profit-maximizer. (One of the many assumptions of perfect competition is profit-maximization by all parties.) Therefore the government may pay economic rents to the owners of resources, i.e., the government pays more than is necessary to attract those resources from alternative uses.

Other deviations from the perfect competition model include monopoly power, externalities, and nonmarginal purchases. In some cases the sellers of resources may possess monopoly power which permits them to obtain economic rents from those operating health programs. An example might be the imposition of regulations requiring the staff of a program to be licensed (as is the case with most health programs). This may severely limit the number of eligible persons and allow them to gain salaries above their opportunity costs.

In the case of externalities, the amount paid to the resource will not reflect the true opportunity costs for society because of unmeasured or unattributable costs. These will be discussed further in Chapter 5.

Finally, there are cases where the purchases made for health programs are so large that they affect the price of the resources being purchased. In these nonmarginal cases the problem is whether the opportunity cost of the resources is equal to their old price, the new price, or a price between the two.

Even with these problems, however, the opportunity costs are assumed to be reflected by the costs of the resources involved. This occurs because no alternative method of valuing foregone opportunities offers a better solution. It is necessary to be cognizant of the possible shortcomings of this approach, however, and to make adjustments when appropriate. (The adjustment is often referred to as "shadow-pricing"-- making an estimate of what the price would have been had a competitive market existed for the sale of the resource.)

Listing of Costs of Health Programs
Obviously, it is important to distinguish whose opportunities are being foregone. We may have the situation where the party who is doing the giving up is not the same as the one who is receiving the benefits. One of the most common mistakes of program evaluation is to ignore the costs incurred by parties other than the government.

Society, individual program clients, health professionals, and the government may each be required to give up resources for participation in the programs. In some cases expenditures of resources will mean foregone opportunities for more than one group. For example, salaries of program administrators will represent costs for society as well as for the government. There will also be resources foregone which will be costs for some groups but which will be gains for other groups. For example, government reimbursements to Medicare or Medicaid program participants or those paid to providers of the services will be costs for the government. Yet, they will actually reduce the costs to the participants and increase the earnings of the providers.[42] Therefore, we once again present separate lists for each party.

A. Costs for Society.
Society's costs for operating health programs consist of the **real** or direct resources (goods and services and not merely funds) which are used up by the program but would have been devoted to other productive uses had the program not occurred. These

---

[42]As a general rule, all changes in resources which occur during the program are considered as costs, and all changes after the program are considered as impacts. There may be gains during the program, such as higher income for the participants, but it is easier to treat these as negative costs.

are the goods and services used in treating the health problem.[43]   Specifically societal costs include:

1. The Time Spent by All Personnel Involved in the Program. Speecial care should be taken to include the time spent by the following groups.   Many are often not considered, particularly those who are not engaged full-time in the program.

   a. Local Center Staff. The costs should include the value of the time they spend on activities such as the design of the grant proposal; marketing services; screening of clients; the provision of any supportive services connected with the program such as education, counseling, custodial care of the equipment and facilities used by the program, day care services, and planning for transportation, diagnosis, direct treatment, therapy, medications supplied; follow-up therapy and counseling; evaluative follow-up; and all of the record keeping and other administrative tasks involved in each of the activities incurred by the program.

   b. Persons at the Regional and State Levels. All persons would be included who are in any way involved in the management, planning, and evaluation of the program. This would include consultants to local health projects, field supervisors, persons responsible for project accreditation and certification, and statisticians involved in

_____

[43]Transfers of funds within society are not societal costs since they do not alter the amount of real resources available only the parties who have use of them.   An example of such transfers are insurance reimbursements.

        reviewing project reports. Again, their salaries should be allocated in proportion to the time spent on the program.

  c. Personnel in the Central Offices of the U.S. Health and Human Services Department or Other Agencies Involved in the Programs. Their salaries should be allocated in proportion to the time spent in administering the program, including budgetary review, fiscal accounting, policy planning, grant approval, project monitoring and evaluation, research, and the training of staff and technical assistants.

2. The Physical Capital Used in the Program. This would include the market rental value of all property, health care equipment, and buildings, including government property, and the market rental value of all equipment and supplies and other materials used in the program. Where market rental value cannot be ascertained, equipment which is purchased should be depreciated based on use. Where it is not possible to estimate depreciation on a use basis, the difference between original cost and salvage value should be amortized appropriately over the life of the program.

3. Miscellaneous Services. All services necessary to the operation of the program, such as staff travel, telephone services and equipment repairs should be measured.

4. The Goods and Services Purchased by the Program Participants Which They Would Not Otherwise Have Bought. This category is particularly relevant to health programs. Costs include such expenditures as transportation to and from the program, out-of-pocket expenses for drugs and other medications, books, and day care for dependents.

5. The Potential Production Which is Lost.

During the time the health care is being
provided, the clients may work less than
they would have worked were they not
involved in the program. This loss of
potential output must be considered a cost
to society. If there are individuals
involved in the operation of the program as
unpaid volunteers, their potential
production during the time they devote to
the program also should be measured. Many
Community Mental Health Centers, for
example, rely heavily on volunteers to
answer phones, provide outreach to clients,
and to participate on citizen advisory
boards.

B. Client/Patient Costs.

These costs include both the direct expenditures
for the health services and treatment received, and
the indirect costs resulting from the impairment.

1. Direct Costs. All payments by the clients
for such program services as diagnosis,
emergency care, treatment, rehabilitation,
and terminal care should be measured.
These include expenditures for hospitalization, outpatient clinical care, nursing
home care, home health care, services of
primary physicians and specialists,
dentists and other professionals, drugs,
rehabilitation counseling and other costs,
such as for prostheses, appliances and
devices to overcome illness-related
impairments, transportation, and other
types of additional care which are not
reimbursed.

2. Indirect Costs. These are the costs
arising when any goods or services are not
produced because people are too ill to work
or keep house because of morbidity or pre-
mature mortality. The measure of output
loss is foregone earnings and the imputed
market value of unperformed housekeeping

services. An adverse effect on productivity can occur if illness lessens the
productivity of persons while on the job;
and absenteeism increases the costs of
production. Indirect costs include the
time spent visiting physicians, unwanted
job changes, and loss of opportunities for
promotion. Illness and disease are also
responsible for a wide variety of psycho-
social deteriorations that are referred to
as social costs. Consequently, victims of
disease may be forced into economic
dependency, social isolation, and other
undesired changes in life plans.

C. Costs for Medical Professionals and Organizations.

Medical professionals often provide unreimbursed
consultation and services to health programs in significant ways, and when they do, those costs should be
calculated. The opportunity costs for medical professionals are those unreimbursed expenditures of health
professionals or organizations devoted to the program
which could have been used for other purposes. These
would include the following expenditures if they are
not offset by reimbursement from insurance companies
or the government.

1. Salaries of Professionals Who Perform
   Services for the Program. The value of
   time devoted to consultation or treatment
   for clients who are not covered by health
   plans, are outside the service area, or are
   not technically eligible for services
   included under the program should be
   included.

2. The Value of All Medical Technology and
   Other Types of Capital Used Up in the
   Program.

3. Miscellaneous Expenditures. Medical professionals and other medical organizations
   may donate goods and services necessary for
   program operation, e.g., drug companies
   provide medications free of charge.

D. Total Government Costs.

Government costs can be viewed in two ways, a) as the total increment in expenditures and reduction in revenues accruing to a unit of government, or b) as the expenditures from a particular line in a budget, labeled for a specific program. The first views the costs from the perspective of the impact on a total government budget. The second takes the perspective of the health program manager. The latter narrower definition of costs is quite simple to measure--it is the amount of funds allocated for the program which has been spent.

The total government cost concept must consider more than the increment in expenditures and use of public resources for the specific program being examined. It must also include the increase or reduction in the use of resources for all other programs which occurs because of the existence of the program under examination. For example, a program manager of a Vocational Rehabilitation (VR) program may try to reduce his or her costs by enrolling illiterate VR clients into an adult basic education program sponsored by the local school system or by CETA rather than by providing the services directly through VR. This will reduce the expenditure of the VR program funds, but the total cost to the government will be the same.

The total government cost concept would examine the following categories of costs for providing services to the participants less the cost of services which would have been provided to the participants in the absence of the program.

1. The Costs of All Personnel for Whom Government Pays the Salaries or Reimburses Others. Personnel to be considered include those discussed in Section A1 and those personnel for whom employers are reimbursed.

2. The Value of All Physical Captial Used in the Program Which is Government Owned or Rented, or for Which Government Reimburses Someone Else.

3. Expenditures on Miscellaneous Services Made
    by Government or for Which Payment is
    Reimbursed by Government.
4. The Net Increase in Government Payments to
    Individuals Made to Induce Them to Engage
    in the Programs.
5. Tax Revenus Lost While Under Treatment.
    These would include the reductions in
    personal income taxes, social security
    taxes and unemployment insurance taxes
    which may result from lower earnings and
    the reductions in sales and excise taxes
    caused by lower expenditures of the clients
    while they are undergoing treatment in a
    program.
6. Other Items for Which Government Makes Pay-
    ments.

Measuring the Increment in Costs

Just as the proper measurement of program impact was
based on the comparison of outcomes with and without
the program, this should also be the key to proper
measurement of program costs. One should consider as
costs only those additional resources that would not
have been used in the absence of the program. For
example, many substance abuse programs involve a job
referral component. When calculating the cost of this
component, the expenditures that the Employment
Service would have made for job referral for these
individuals if the program had not existed must be
subtracted from the program expenditure on this
item. Only if this subtraction is made will the
increment in the resources used by the program be
calculated, and it is only this concept which can be
compared with the measures of additional well-being
which were discussed earlier.
    Thus, to measure many of the costs requires know-
ledge of what would have happened to the program
clients had they not participated. What would happen,
for example, if the alcoholics, heroin addicts,
sexually active adolescents, young mothers had not
received special health services? The best way to get

this knowledge is to use a control group which is randomly selected from persons willing and able to enter the program. Only this group will give an internally valid estimate. Thus if costs are to be as accurately estimated as program outcomes the same type of control group must be used to measure both. If projects are selected for evaluation when funded, this will permit the same control groups to be used to measure the costs and impacts of a program.

The Use of Control Groups. Control groups should be used to provide information for three types of cost estimates. The first is the loss incurred while the clients receive services from the program. While participating in some programs, individuals may not be engaged in what they normally would be doing. Therefore, participation in the program may lead to losses of after tax earnings, unemployment compensation, or welfare payments by the individuals; potential production by society; and taxes by government. The experience of the control group during the course of the program, however, should not be affected by the program. Therefore, the difference between the control group members' and participants' after tax earnings, unemployment compensation, welfare payments, production, and taxes will show the losses actually incurred because of participation in the program.

The second use of control groups is to determine how much of the governmental services received by the participants would not have been received if there had been no program. Earlier we discussed Employment Service job referral services which would otherwise be used by many of the persons who enter substance abuse programs. Similarly, when Medicare or Medicaid recipients enter such programs the treatment or therapy they receive in the program may merely replace treatment or therapy they would have received elsewhere. Therefore, it is important that information be collected on the amount and nature of all services received by both the participants and the control group. If this is known, the latter can be subtracted from the former to find the actual increment in services which result from a program. Then, only the cost of this increment in services should be compared

with the benefits which were calculated as the
differences between the two groups.[44]

Finally, the control group can be used to measure
the increment in program-related expenditures by the
participants. Some programs require that those
receiving services incur expenses for travel, drugs
and other medical tests, living expenses and meals
away from home, etc. Some of these expenditures
represent added costs of program participation; however, others may not. If an individual would be
taking the bus to work instead of taking it to a
health care center were he or she not in a program,
there may be no additional cost of transportation
resulting from the program. To arrive at this
conclusion it is necessary to know the expenditures
associated with the program by the participants and
the expenditures on these items by the control group.

If it is not possible to have a control group, the
same information should be gathered for a comparison
group. All of the same internal validity problems
will occur in the measurement of costs as were discussed with reference to benefits in Chapter 3. Therefore, once again we strongly reiterate our recommenda-
tion that control groups be used.

Measuring Costs for Other Family Members. In
addition to the control group, measurements should
also be made for other persons who might be affected
by the program. One group which is very likely to be
affected is the client's family. For instance, if
participation in an alcohol treatment abuse program
lowers the earnings of the participant, the slack may

---

[44]The implicit assumption in the use of a control
group to measure the increment in services is that the
level of service provided by the program being
evaluated does not alter the amount of service
provided by other programs. In terms of the examples
the funding of additional Vocational Rehabilitation
programs should not reduce the amount of the
Employment Service or public assistance case worker
aid provided to the control group.

be taken up by another family member who accepts a temporary job which he or she would not normally have taken. Illness can also force a family to incur expenses in caring and providing for the sick member of the family. Such changes could be discovered by comparing the work experiences during the program, not only of the participants and members of the control groups, but also of their respective families.

Accurately Measuring the Costs

Government accounting systems are designed on an appropriations basis and not on the basis of incremental costs. Typical government cost accounting says that anything paid out in the name of a program is a cost of that program. As a result, many items are improperly charged to a program while other costs are ignored. Some specific examples of these problems follow.

Proper Program Assignment. The costs of functions performed for a program sometimes are not charged to that program. We have already discussed the example where medical professionals sometimes work overtime without charging the program, while other times they may be fully reimbursed. Under present accounting procedures these costs are all assigned to the program in the latter case and all assigned to the professional in the former. Yet the same services are being performed for the program participants in the two areas. Other examples of costs that are often improperly assigned are health education, which is sometimes provided by the local public health department; the use of hospital facilities and equipment for inpatient services; the time spent by various public officials preparing project proposals; and the value of the services of volunteers or of persons on loan from medical education institutions.[45] Therefore, in

_____

[45]Valuing the opportunity cost of volunteers' time is especially difficult because the volunteers may be using leisure time. A truly satisfactory method for

these and many other institutions one must go beyond the costs directly assigned to a program in order to include the costs of all of the additional services provided because individuals participate in a program.

Similarly, if expenditures are assigned to one program but in fact are made in part for other programs, only a portion of their costs should be included. For instance, equipment purchased for one program subsequently may be used for others (such as diagnostic machines bought by a hospital which are subsequently used to train health professionals), or persons who are hired for one project may also be used on other projects.

Inclusion of All Costs. All of the costs of a program should be measured. Yet, there are several items frequently overlooked. The first, the value of public facilities provided free of charge, was discussed above. While the use of these facilities does not represent an outlay of funds, there are still costs involved. Most equipment will wear out with use, and their use by health programs will accelerate the need for replacement or repair. Therefore, the depreciation of this equipment should be calculated and included in the costs of the programs. This will be particularly important for the often quite expensive diagnostic equipment which may become scientifically obsolete even before it mechanically deteriorates.

Even for buildings that will suffer little from the additional wear, there are still costs associated with their use by health programs. Other activities may be displaced. For instance, if a high school auditorium is used for hypertension screening, school functions may have to be held elsehwere or may not be held at all. Both of these alternatives will involve costs. Similarly, even when an unused public building is reactivated and used as a store front clinic there are

---

assigning a dollar value to leisure has yet to be developed. Presumably, it is at least as valuable as the income the individual could earn were he or she employed (if leisure is less valuable the person would go to work).

costs if the property could have been sold or leased to private industry. Thus, to measure the true cost of these facilities, they should be valued at their market rental value.

The administrative cost of health programs is another category typically underreported. There is a large administrative overhead connected with each program. The time that civil servants at the national and regional levels spend on planning the original program, project review and monitoring, program-connected evaluation and research, fiscal appropriations and accounting, and on all other administrative duties should be considered. Ideally, the time spent by all government workers from the Secretary of Health and Human Services on down should be apportioned among programs and among particular projects, if possible. Greater attempts should be made to approximate the services provided in each of these categories since they represent sizeable costs which presently are excluded from most calculations.

Calculating Marginal Costs

Another important concept for measuring both impacts and costs is that they should be measured at the margin. Health programs are evaluated for the most part in order to say whether they should be expanded or contracted rather than whether they should be maintained at their present size or eliminated. Therefore, what is needed are the benefits and costs associated with various changes in their size. For instance, what will be the difference in total benefits and costs of immunizing 5,000 additional persons for an innoculation program? Often the cost of providing additional services is considerably below the average cost for an existing program. For example, the cost of immunizing additional people may be insignificant since the facility, vaccine, and health professionals are already committed. The result is a declining cost curve such that the marginal cost is considerably below the average cost and the benefit-cost ratio at the margin is much higher than it is on the average (assuming constant benefits).

Yet, generally only overall costs and benefits are considered and not those at the margin. Only if the ratio of average benefits and costs is proportionate to benefits and costs at the margin for all programs will average calculations of benefits and costs be accurate guides for making program decisions. The problem, however, is how to measure benefits and costs at the margin.

One way of looking at the problem is in terms of the total national program. If it has had a long history and has operated at a number of different sizes there may be a sufficient total number of points to construct a total cost curve; the first derivative of that curve will yield the marginal cost of the program. One can similarly calculate marginal benefits. This procedure requires a number of different studies over a broad range of program services and program sizes. Unfortunately, the real world operation of health programs does not usually lend itself to this type of analysis because many of the programs have been recently developed or modified.

Another method of calculating marginal cost is based upon the costs of providing services in programs of various sizes at the local level. In this situation, health services providers are the unit of observation. Arraying providers by size and cost per service will show the marginal cost of additional service. This procedure, however, has a potential limitation stemming from the possible correlation between the size of the program and the health-related environmental conditions in which it exists. Thus, a program of 500 participants in New York City may yield costs that are quite different than a program of 500 in Pottsville, New York.

Joint Costs

Joint costs exist when the use of resources produces more than one type of output. The classic example is the raising of sheep to produce both mutton and wool. In this situation, once the sheep have been raised for wool there is no additional cost to raising them for mutton. Or alternatively, once raised for

mutton there is no additional cost to having them
produce wool. An example of a joint cost in the
health field is when staff are shared between more
than one organizational unit, or two or more organizations such as in a teaching hospital where the
training of students also yields health services to
the patients. The question is, "When a resource is to
be used for one of these purposes, should any cost be
assigned to the other purpose?" Some people argue
that since the primary goal of a teaching hospital is
to produce health professionals, there is no need to
charge any costs to the hospital since the marginal
cost of that service is zero. While such logic is
true for sheep's wool and mutton, it is not true for
the type of health services being discussed.
Presumably, the students' services would be available
to some other health facility, who might pay for their
services.

Examining the Costs of the First Program Clients

The cost of a particular program will vary, depending
on when in the course of the program's development the
measurement is made. As with most businesses, the
costs of health programs will decline as their size
and duration increase. A program will have relatively
high costs per clients when it is being developed and
the number of clients is small. Program staff will be
engaged in training personnel, establishing bookkeep-
ing systems, writing proposals or marketing services,
experimenting with program ideas, and organizing
related services. As the program becomes more established and experience is gained, less time will be
spent on these activities and more time can be devoted
to providing services, increasing the number of participants, and reducing unit costs.   While the benefits

may not change with program size,[46] it is almost certain that the program costs will change. Therefore, the time period in which the costs of a program are measured will be crucial, particularly at the beginning of a program.

To resolve the problem for a new program, we suggest that the benefits of the first program clients should be related to the costs for later clients in the program.[47] While this would cause the costs assigned to the first group of program clients to be below those actually incurred, it would give a better indication of the long run costs of the program after it has become more established. Moreover, it would not lead to any delay in evaluation since, as has been mentioned, the success of the program should not be measured until one year after clients received the health care services, or leave the program.[48]

---

[46]It is possible that benefit levels will also change as the program develops. This could occur if as the program managers devote more time to providing services the quality of such services improves.

[47]Cost data still should be gathered at the start of the program to make comparisons with latter cost figures, to find the extent of decline in costs with increases in the size of the program, and for administrative purposes.

[48]In view of the difficulties involved in comparing the results of various health program evaluations, the Public Health Service recently published a set of recommended guidelines for conducting such studies. See Hodgson and Meiners (80).

Exercise 4-1

The following table lists the costs for operation of a 6 month program to manage stress, and counsel spouses who are newly separated. It is sponsored jointly by a federally funded community health and mental health center. Fees are on a sliding scale basis depending on a person's income. Under this program clients spend half the time participating in seminars and half the time practicing stress reducing exercises. A weekend marathon session is planned midway through the program. At the top of each column are the parties who might incur the costs. Place a (+) in the box if positive costs are incurred, a minus (-) if negative costs are incurred (i.e., if the party receives resources instead of losing them), and a zero (0) if there are no costs to the party.

Parties Bearing Costs

Type of Expense	Society	Govern-ment	Health Pro-fessionals and Organizations	Client
I. Center Expenses A. Personnel—salary, fringe benefits and value of payment in kind made to: 1. Therapists, group leaders, and other types of instructors				

Type of Expense	Parties Bearing Costs			
	Society	Government	Health Professionals and Organizations	Client
2. Administrators (center directors, clinical directors, etc.)				
3. Other institution personnel (janitors, clerical and book-keeping personnel)				
4. Administrators outside the institution (planners, administrators of the program at the local and regional levels)				
B. Supplies and materials used as part of the therapy process				
C. Transporation costs paid to the clients				

Type of Expense	Parties Bearing Costs			
	Society	Government	Health Professionals and Organizations	Client
D. Space and equipment				
E. Fees received as compensation for the course (1) from the government (2) from clients (3) from other sources				
II. Earnings Foregone A. Expected earnings of the clients were they not in treatment				
B. Value of the services of volunteers who aid clinics were they to be purchased				

Parties Bearing Costs

Type of Expense	Society	Government	Health Professionals and Organizations	Client
C. Taxes which are not paid because of reduced earnings (1) by clients while in the program, (2) by volunteers while in the program				
III. Student Out-of-Pocket Expense A. Reading materials				
B. Transportation to the center				
C. Expenses for room or board during the weekend marathon				
D. Fees, if charged				

Suggested Readings

Averill, R., et al. "A Cost-Benefit Analysis of Continued Stay Certification," Medical Care 15, February 1977.

Bunker, J.P., ed. Costs, Risks, and Benefits of Surgery, New York, NY: Oxford University Press, 1977.

Cretin, S. "Cost-Benefit Analysis of Treatment and Prevention of Myocardial Infarction," Health Services Research, 12, Summer 1977.

Doherty, N., et al. "Cost-Effectiveness Analysis and Alternative Health Care Programs for the Elderly," Health Services Research, 12, Summer 1977.

Grosse, R. "Cost-Benefit Analysis of Health Services," Annals of the American Academy of Political and Social Science, 399, January 1972.

Luce, B. "Allocating Costs and Benefits in Disease Prevention Programs: An Application to Cervical Cancer Screening," in The Implications of Cost-Effectiveness Analysis of Medical Technology, "Background Paper #2: Case Studies of Medical Technologies," prepared at the Office of Technology Asssessment, U.S. Congress, Washington, D.C., 1980.

Neuhauser, D., and Lewicki, A. "What Do We Gain from the Sixth Stool Guaiac?" New England Journal of Medicine, 293, July 31, 1975.

COMBINING THE MEASURES OF PROGRAM IMPACT AND COST

The data gathered for evaluations of health programs should provide the information to answer four types of questions. (1) Should a particular program or service be continued? (2) Which of several alternative programs should be expanded or contracted? (3) In what ways can changes in the services provided by a particular program lead to improved efficiency? (4) What services or programs best serve particular groups of individuals? The data discussed in the previous chapters will provide the answers to these questions. Before such answers can be obtained, however, several technical decisions must be made. These include: how to handle potential impacts which occur after measurement, how to treat impacts and costs which occur over time, and how to handle external effects and secondary impacts.

Treating Future Impacts [49]

Health programs may affect the clients for the remainder of their lives. Therefore, to accurately assess all of the impacts of these programs it would be desirable to wait until all persons in the program have died.[50]   Obviously such a suggestion is ludicrous. The purpose of program evaluation is to make policy decisions on whether the program or services should be continued, and if so, in what form and for whom. The decision maker cannot wait 20 or more years

---

[49]We concentrate on questions relating to impacts since we have defined all effects, positive or negative, which occur after the program as impacts and those which occur during the program as costs. Most of the impacts after the program should involve positive benefits.

[50]Since there may also be intergenerational effects, an even longer period of observation may be needed.

before he or she makes a judgment. We have suggested that the measurement of impacts should occur one year after the provision of the health services. This will require estimating what impacts will occur after these measurements are made. Such estimation requires two sets of projections: how will program impacts change over time and how long will the impacts last?

How the Impacts Might Occur Over Time. It is conceivable that the impacts of a health program might grow, remain constant, or decline as time passes. For the individual receiving health care services they might grow to the extent that he or she is able to achieve a new and higher occupational level by virtue of an improvement in health status. A good example here would be the vocational rehabilitation program which provides artificial limbs. Most of this program's clients would have little expected earnings during the rest of their lifetimes in the absence of extensive prosthetic treatment, physical therapy, and vocational training. With the training and the prosthetic devices they are able to function, at least partially, in the employment world and to receive the earnings' increases most people usually receive as they build seniority.

Alternatively, one can see situations where the effect of a health program might lead to constant benefits. An individual who might have died is saved through dialysis, emergency care, or rehabilitation practices. Benefits accrue both to the recipient and to his or her family for the amount of life saved as a result of the health program.

Finally, there may be a situation where the impacts of the health program decline as time passes. This may be due either to the re-emergence of the disease or illness, or a decline in the practices of good health habits. Examples of the former are where effects of immunizations decrease over time and the clients need to be reimmunized or become vulnerable to the disease. Similarly the former participants of an alcohol detoxification and counseling center may fail to remain continent over an extended time period. In these cases the initial advantages provided to clients may be eliminated with the passage of time.

Given these possible divergent streams of inputs over time, which one is appropriate? The most logical method for making projections would be to base them on the experience of other clients in the program. If the gains for a similar program have led to health benefits that might be translated into monetary gains of five percent, then this figure could be applied. Unfortunately, there is no absolutely reliable basis for comparison. Most cost-benefit evaluations are less than ten years old, and the data base from longitudinal studies is insufficient to make realistic projections at this time.

The Duration of Impacts. If it is found that the gains of program participation decline steadily over time they may eventually reach zero.[51] Alternatively, if they remain constant or increase during the period of observation, they may continue until the individual dies. The magnitude of the project impacts and the resulting program evaluation will be greatly affected by which of these scenarios is selected and by how far into the future the projections are made. Different studies have chosen one or the other alternative.

A Possible Solution. The best method for estimating future impacts appears to us to be a sensitivity analysis which projects the impacts for several periods with the impacts increasing, remaining constant, and declining. A matrix can be constructed which presents the expected impacts under each of the alternatives (e.g., Table 5-1). Such a matrix will show the sensitivity of the impact estimates to various combinations of assumptions, which should be useful when comparing different programs or services.

As longitudinal studies provide more hard data on the trends in impacts over time, the matrix can be condensed. Until then, considerable thought should be given to determining which description of the particular impact studied is most appropriate. Filling in the matrix is only the first step in projecting

---

[51]Longer term projections should also take mortality rates into account.

Table 5-1

Total Impacts Under Alternative Assumptions

Period of Impact Life	Impacts Decline Annually by:		Impacts are Constant	Impacts Increase Annually by:	
	5%	15%		5%	15%
5 Years					
10 Years					
20 Years					
Over 20 Years					

impacts--theoretical or empirical considerations for selecting the "best estimate" must follow.

Assigning Values to Future Impacts and Costs

The benefits of different types of health programs may be realized over different periods of time. Likewise, various impacts of a program occur at different points in time following treatment. Finally, program impacts occur in the future (after treatment), whereas costs are incurred in the present (during treatment). The basic question to be answered is "Are impacts to be treated equally regardless of when they occur; if they are not, what is the proper method for equating future impacts with those which occur now or costs which have reimbursements. already been incurred?"[52]

To construct a simple example, take three medical procedures that require an investment in 1983 of 80 million dollars for technology and support services. Procedure A will return 80 million dollars in 1984 from fees and other type benefits for the clients. Program B will return 40 million dollars of fees and other type benefits for the clients in 1984, 40 million dollars of benefits in 1985, and 40 million dollars of benefits in 1986. Thereafter, there will be no benefits. Program C will provide benefits of 20 million dollars for each of the seven years from 1984 through 1990, after which there will be no benefits. Which program is preferable, or are all three unacceptable?

Program A is unlikely to be the choice because most people are not indifferent toward options giving them an equal amount of benefits now and in the future. This occurs for two related reasons. The first of these is "time preference." This is the old saying, "A bird in the hand is worth two in the bush." Simple proof of this desire to have our cake now rather than in the future is that most of us require that we be paid a certain amount in order for us to postpone consumption. In order for the bank to induce us to make deposits, they must make interest payments. Similarly, most people borrow money and pay interest in order to buy things now rather than to wait until they have the necessary cash for the purchase. Individuals will pay fifteen percent interest charges in order to have a new car now rather than saving the money and buying it two years from now. The individual's rate of time preference, which is subjective, can be estimated by his or her willingness to loan or to borrow. He or she will loan money as long as the

---

[52]Increasingly in the literature effectiveness measures are being discounted. Stange and Sumner (135) as well as Weinstein and Stason (151) discounted effectiveness measures of mortality avoided in the future.

return is greater than his or her time preference rate and will borrow money as long as the interest rate paid is less than this time preference rate.[53]

Another way of looking at the problem of valuing future benefits in terms of present expenditures is in terms of the opportunity cost of alternative projects. If a person can earn interest of 6 percent by putting money into a riskless savings account, he or she would be foolish to invest in a project which paid less than six percent. Similar logic applies to government projects. The government should not undertake any project which pays less than the alternative investments that it might undertake or the return the resources would earn in the private sector.[54] The use of private sector rates of return is important because taxation of the private sector is the source of the resources which will be used to undertake the project.

The two concepts are interrelated. In a perfectly competitive capital market, as borrowers whose time preference is high borrow more, the interest rate will rise and their time preference will fall. Similarly, the interest rates lenders can charge will fall and their time preference will rise as they choose the best of alternative projects. Eventually, an equilibrium point will be reached where the borrowing rate, the loan rate, the rate of time preference, and the opportunity cost of alternative projects will be

---

[53]It must be recognized that there are factors other than time preference--such as precautionary saving for a rainy day--which will influence willingness to borrow and loan at various interest rates.

[54]This statement holds only if the returns from the projects are fully and accurately measured. It may be that the government project has certain noneconomic benefits which are socially desirable and which cannot be expressed in economic terms. In this case, the government project might be undertaken even though it does not yield the rate of return attainable in the private market.

equal. This will be "the" discount rate--the rate by which future returns would have to be reduced to find their present value. The formula for determining the present value of impacts is:

$$PV_B = \frac{B_1}{(1+r)} + \frac{B_2}{(1+r)^2} + \dots \frac{B_n}{(1+r)^n} = \sum_{t=1}^{n} \frac{B_t}{(1+r)^t}$$

where B_1, B_2, B_n are the benefits (net of losses) in years 1, 2, and n, respectively; r is the rate of discount; and t is the year. In terms of our example, if the discount rate is ten percent, the present value of the benefits of the three programs are 72.7 million dollars for Program A, 99.5 million dollars for Program B, and 97.4 million dollars for Program C.

Unfortunately, in the real world the capital market is not perfect. There are several major factors which prevent the establishment of a single discount rate. One is the tax rate on private projects. Since the corporate profit rate approaches 50 percent, a project needs to have a rate of return at least twice as high as the individual's rate of time preference in order for the project to be worthwhile to undertake. Another consideration would be that projects are not equally risky. An individual in making his or her calculation of the rate of return must include some premium for the risk involved in the project. Therefore, the rate of return may have to exceed the rate of time preference before it will be worthwhile for the individual to undertake a project. Furthermore, the rate of risk will vary among projects so that there will be a whole variety of interest rates charged to arrive at an equally riskless rate of return. Other disrupting factors which will lead to a diversion of interest rates from the single discount rate will be various market imperfections, such as lack of communication, imperfect knowledge, monopolies, and outright discrimination. Finally, there is a problem of externalities in that the rate of return in the private market may not take into account all of the costs or the benefits which are derived from the project. This is a problem of proper allocation of costs and returns to a project. For instance, the owners of a polluting smokestack may not be charged for the pollution. The pollution exists, however, and it lowers the rate of return on the project for society although it does not lower the private rate of return. In conclusion, there is not a single discount rate which can automatically be applied to all health projects, services, and technologies.

Which rate, then, should be used? [55]   As stated above, the discount rate should be no lower than the amount people are willing to pay to borrow funds to increase consumption nor should it be less than the return the funds could earn in alternative investments. These rates differ, however, depending on who is borrowing and who is investing. The government borrowing rate, practically risk free to the lender, has recently been between 4 and 15 percent. Business faces a somewhat higher rate--the prime rate has been between 6 and 22 percent in recent years. Individuals face many borrowing rates ranging from about 8 percent to over 25 percent depending on the risk involved to the lender. The alternative investment opportunities also vary. The basic alternative to a government program is a tax cut which will allow increases in private business investment. The real return on private investment is in the range of 10 to 20 percent, part of which is a premium for risk. The return to the individual is typically lower (5 to 15 percent), again dependent on the risk involved. Since the extent of risk is not known in the investment cases, the true rate of return is not known for alternative projects.

To quote Prest and Turvey (111) "the truth of the matter is that, whatever one does, one is trying to unscramble an omelette, and no one has yet invented a uniquely superior way of doing this." Therefore, the

---

[55]The Office of Management and Budget in 1972 set a rate of ten percent. The ten percent rate represented an average rate of return in the private sector before taxes and after inflation.

most logical way to proceed is to consider a variety
of possible discount rates and then to test how sen-
sitive the analysis is to each choice. Rates of 5
percent, 10 percent, 15 percent, and 20 percent would
appear to represent a reasonable set. They should
cover the range of time preference rates. For most
health program comparisons, the relative values of the
impacts of two services will vary little with the
choice of discount rate. In some situations, however,
substantially different results will occur.[56]

If only a single discount rate is to be used, it
would appear that the consensus is now at a rate of
ten percent, particularly for discounting society's
future benefits. This rate roughly approximates the
return on private investment when a small allowance is
made for risk. However, other rates should be used as
well in order to demonstrate the sensitivity of the
analysis to this assumption.

Accounting for Externalities

Up to this point, governmental and societal impacts
and costs basically have been calculated by aggregat-
ing the impacts and costs associated with the program
clients. We must now be concerned with external
impacts and costs--benefits and costs accruing to
persons who are not directly participating in the
health program.

The question may be raised as to why these outside
individuals should be considered. The answer is that
these individuals may be affected in ways that completely offset any value of the program. If children
in the health program are vaccinated, and prevented
from contracting a disease, other children in the

---

[56]In terms of our example a five percent discount rate
will cause Program C to be preferable, whereas Program
B has the highest yield using a rate of ten percent.
If an 80 percent rate is used, Program A is the best
of the three alternatives but no program would be
preferred to all three.

community may also not catch the disease. Or consider
a training program for allied health professionals.
It is conceivable that program participants are placed
in jobs which would have gone to other individuals had
the program not existed. Further, it is possible that
the program participants replaced individuals with
identical characteristics so that there is no net
increase in employment in the aggregate or for any
particular group in society. Alternatively, the program participants may replace other individuals who
hold political power with the result that the program
becomes politically infeasible because the latter
refuse to allow the program to exist. Similar issues
revolve around the question of who pays the costs of
health programs.

Measuring the Externalities.[57]   By definition,
externalities are difficult to measure. They require
identification of the parties outside the program and
the comparison of their situations in the presence of
the program with what would have happened in its
absence. For members of the participants' families
such procedures are relatively easy--the families of
control or comparison group members will represent the
situation without the program.

The other externalities do not lend themselves to
these measurements. There is no way to identify
positively the individuals who would have contracted a
disease or illness were the program clients not
treated. The best that appears possible is to realize

---

[57]There are two types of external benefits and costs,
real and pecuniary. Real externalities involve the
creation of additional real production (real goods and
services which would not have existed before), or they
use additional real resources (and therefore they
reduce the amounts of goods and services which can be
produced). The real external effects are particularly
important when one is discussing the impacts and costs
of health programs from society's point of view.
Pecuniary externalities affect incomes but not
resource use or creation.

that the externalities are dependent on the overall health of a nation and the size of the program.

Secondary Impacts. In the preceding section the discussion concerned direct effects of health programs on persons external to the programs. There may also be indirect effects of the spending for the programs-- the secondary or multiplier effects of the programs. In its simplest form, the logic runs as follows. Health programs represent an increment in expenditures. As the monies for the program are spent on the program clients, this will lead to greater income for other individuals who receive the funds. These individuals will, in turn, spend more. The expenditures will cause increases in production through the multiplier effect. These secondary effects could also be included among the impacts of the program.

Most evaluations, however, ultimately concern the choice of alternative program expenditures or a reduction in taxes. These alternatives will also have secondary effects, and it becomes merely a question of how the multiplier will be called into effect and not whether it will be applicable. Since all programs will have a multiplier effect, there seems no point in considering it directly. One need not multiply the benefits by a fixed factor (such as a multiplier of two or three) since all programs will presumably have such a multiplier.[58]

Making Program Decisions

In Chapter 2 we outlined a series of many different types of possible criteria for measuring program

---

[58]An argument can be made that the size of the multiplier will vary depending on the type of expenditure and how it is used. Also, government expenditures may have a higher multiplier than a tax cut. Estimating the magnitudes of the differences, however, is not practical and, therefore, the multipliers are probably best ignored.

impacts.   Any or all of these criteria may be
considered to be important by a decision maker
evaluating a program. Therefore, a measure of program
impact and cost should be calculated for every
criterion which has been examined in the analysis.
   Combinations of Program Impact and Cost Measures.
The basic tools for combining measures of program
impact and cost are benefit-cost and cost-effectiveness ratios.[59]   These express the total or average
amount of success (net of losses) per dollar of
cost.   Further, since the benefits and costs occur at
different times the ratio should show the present
value of each, i.e.,

$$\frac{\text{Present value of benefits}}{\text{Present value of costs}} = \frac{\sum\limits_{t=1}^{n} B_t/(1+r)^t}{\sum\limits_{t=1}^{n} C_t/(1+r)^t}$$

where B_t and C_t are the benefits and costs for each
year in which they occur, r is the discount rate, and
t is the year. Usually, both terms in the ratio will
be positive.   This indicates that while the program
produces benefits it involves the use of resources to
accomplish this gain.   When a benefit-cost ratio is
greater than one, it indicates that the present value
of the economic returns exceeds the present value of
the costs of the program. If the ratio is less than
one, this indicates that the program costs more than
the value of the resources gained from it.   For

---

[59]The expression is a benefit-cost ratio when the
criteria of success are measured in dollars (such as
increases in a client's earnings) so that the numerator and the denominator are expressed in dollar
terms. If the numerator is expressed in a unit other
than dollars (such as number of persons treated or
change in score on a quality of life scale), the
expression is a cost-effectiveness ratio.

noneconomic gains, a subjective weighting is necessary.

Whereas the benefit-cost ratio is probably the most widely used criterion for evaluating projects, it suffers from several possible shortcomings. First, as discussed earlier, the benefits of many medical procedures, health services, and programs are not clearly known. This approach is most reliable, then, for outcomes of treatment which are quantifiable in monetary terms. Many of the intangible benefits resulting from improved health are difficult to quantify in monetary terms, and others cannot be quantified.

The issue of how to determine the economic value of a life saved as a result of health services is particularly critical. One method is to use the present value of the future stream of income--the livelihood-savings approach.[60]

Another alternative is the "willingness to pay" approach. It is the sum of the amounts individuals are willing to pay for the reduction in health risk attributable to a life-saving program or medical procedure. What, for example, would an alcoholic, or his or her family, be willing to pay to be rehabilitated?

Studies that compare the efficiency of life enhancing programs should also compare days involving limited activity. This can be accomplished by connecting limited activity days to some fraction of healthy days. If, for example, we were to determine the value of life saved for a person through help of dialysis support, we would ask the persons to equate healthy days with days of life with dialysis. If the person agrees that they are half as valuable, we would weight each life saved by dialysis by .5. It is recognized that it is probably impossible to value the benefits received relative to the relief of many ailments, such as upper respiratory tract infections,

---

[60]See Cooper and Rice (49) and Georgetown University (67). The reader is also referred to the earlier discussion in Chapter 2 of the present volume.

headaches, vaginitis, etc. In such cases, global impacts, e.g., measures relating to quality of life, satisfaction with health care, days no longer absent from work, may be applied in assessing the benefits.[61]

Secondly, if either term in the benefit-cost ratio is negative there are problems of interpretation. A negative numerator and a positive denominator indicate that not only are the original costs never recovered, but in addition, further losses are incurred after the conclusion of the program. On the other hand, if the numerator is positive and the denominator is negative, the program not only generates successful outcomes on its completion but also provides more resources during the program than it consumes. If both the numerator and denominator are negative the net gains are generated during the period of the program while net losses occur after the completion of the program. Such a situation is highly unusual.

A related problem with benefit-cost ratios is that one must be clear as to what constitutes a benefit and what constitutes a cost. Earlier, we suggested that costs include those changes which occur during the course of the program of treatment and that impacts are any changes which occur after the end of the program or treatment. However, because different treatments occur over different periods, it becomes somewhat difficult to apply the definitions of benefits and costs equally to all programs and treatments.

---

[61]See Kane, et al (88). The authors developed a practical method for determining the functional outcome status of patients in an ambulatory setting. The levels used were: (1) the patient performs usual major activity; (2) performs usual major activity but has abnormal laboratory test or physical finding; (3) performs usual major activity and is symptomatic; (4) has cut down on major activity; (5) limited in ability; (6) bed disabled; (7) death. Certain cost estimates might be placed on each of these functional outcome states based on the client's "willingness to pay" or restored earning power.

A third problem with the benefit-cost ratio is that it requires that a rate of discount be established to find the present value of the benefits and costs. As discussed earlier, the selection of a particular discount rate may be subject to question, particularly since the choice of rate may determine the magnitude of the benefit-cost ratio. However, one does have the opportunity to make a sensitivity analysis to find out how the benefit-cost ratios for different projects and interventions vary in their ranking if different discount rates are used. When such differences occur, another combination of benefits and costs may be more appropriate.

When the numerator or the denominator of a benefit-cost ratio is negative or there are substantial problems in differentiating benefits and costs, another combination of impact and cost measures--the net present value which gives the net value of the gain from the program--is usually more appropriate. This may be expressed as:

The present value of benefits minus the present value of costs
or

$$\sum_{t=1}^{n} B_t/(1+r)^t - \sum_{t=1}^{n} C_t/(1+r)^t$$

It shows the present value of the additional resources which have been gained after costs have been deducted. Therefore, the net present value must exceed zero in order for the program to cover its costs.

While the net present value combination solves the problems of negative costs or benefits and the definition of benefits and costs, it, too, suffers shortcomings. These include the problem of choosing a discount rate. In addition, it should be obvious that the net present value can only be calculated when both the benefits and costs are expressed in the same units, as is also true for benefit-cost ratios. One cannot subtract apples from oranges or dollars from units gained on a satisfaction scale. Also, when comparing alternative programs for achieving similar outcomes, the net present value is appropriate only when the expenditures on the alternatives can be the same.

A third measure, when both the numerator and denominator are expressed in dollars, is the internal rate of return. This is the annual discount rate which will equate the total benefits and costs. To estimate the rate of return the following equation is solved for r:

$$\sum_{t=1}^{n} \left(\frac{B_t}{(1+r)^t} - \frac{C_t}{(1+r)^t} \right) = 0$$

For a program to be successful, it must have a return greater than zero. To be better than an alternative program, it must have a higher rate than does the alternative.

The obvious advantage of the internal rate of return approach over the others is that it does not require an explicit discount rate and thus avoids the problem of choosing one. Also, it makes no difference whether a particular change is labeled as a negative benefit or a positive cost. The internal rate of return suffers, however, from other shortcomings. Most important of these is that it cannot be calculated without the use of computer facilities.

Should Health Services or Programs be Continued? The answer to this question usually depends on what alternative treatments or services are available. General agreement should exist on the discontinuation of certain types of services or programs. A service or program should be ended when no redeeming features are found after consideration of all criteria of success; that is, where all important dependent variables are measured and: (1) no benefit-cost ratio is greater than one, and (2) no cost-effectiveness ratio has a positive numerator or a negative denominator. These criteria will be met very infrequently if only because it is usually impossible to quantify all of the dependent variables. Therefore, the program decisions must be based on a comparison of alternative interventions or services.

Comparison of Alternative Programs.   In very few cases one program is superior to another when compared on all of the criteria that we have suggested.   In these cases the course of action is clear; the superior program should be expanded. (This is based on the assumption that average benefits and costs are positively related to those at the margin.)   More often, one finds a program will be superior in some areas but inferior in others. The choice of program expansion and contraction under these circumstances depends upon the preferences attached to each of the benefits.   For example, a coronary rehabilitation program may be more effective than a preventive health program in raising the life expectancy of the partici-pants, but the preventive program may lead to an overall healthier life style and a reduction in aggre-gate health care costs.[62]   Assuming that only one program can be expanded, a choice must be made as to which is more important--increased life expectancy or

---

[62]So far the discussion has concentrated on the econo-mic benefits, where the numerator can be expressed in dollars.   Although noneconomic benefits cannot be stated in comparable terms, it is extremely important that these benefits not be ignored.   It is useful, therefore, to present the noneconomic cost-effective-ness ratios in tabular form for the decision maker to use along with the economic data. These will take the form of ratios of the increment in a noneconomic benefit divided by the cost of achieving that incre-ment.   For instance, a dialysis program may increase the client's personal satisfaction by two points on a scale of 20 at a cost of $50. The ratio then would be 1:25.   The fact that it may be done at home, rather than in a hospital, might increase the personal satisfaction by one point for a cost of $100 for a ratio of 1:100.   It will then be up to the decision maker to assign relative weights to the benefit-cost ratio and to each of the cost-effectiveness ratios.

psychic improvements and reduction in health costs.
Once explicit weights showing relative importance are
assigned to each of these impacts, the program
decisions can be made. The weights should be explicit
so that others who have different values can also use
the analysis.

There are two strategies which may be followed in
assigning relative weights to program impacts. The
first is for the decision maker to provide the evaluator with the weights of various benefits before the
evaluation is begun. The evaluator will then examine
only those measures of success with nonzero weights
and will aggregate his or her findings to arrive at a
single overall measure of program effectiveness. The
advantage of this approach is that it does not
consider goals deemed irrelevant (those given no
weight by the decision maker); therefore, it may be
more economical and efficient. Its major shortcoming
is that the weights assigned to impacts differ among
decision makers and over time. For this reason the
alternative approach usually is more practical.

In the second strategy the evaluator calculates the
benefit-cost or cost-effectiveness ratio for every
impact which might be relevant for each program or
service being examined. If consideration of all
possible impacts is not possible because of cost or
other limitations, the calculations should at least be
made for all impacts which are thought highly relevant. The ratios for alternative programs or services
can then be compared in a single table, such as Table
5-2. This procedure allows each decision maker to
assign the weights that he or she believes are most
appropriate and to arrive at a decision of overall
value. If circumstances change, the decision maker
can redefine the weights and simply recalculate the
relative performance of the health services. The
weights should be determined independently of the
results of the analysis; otherwise, there is a great
postanalysis temptation to find the weights which will
make the analytical results conform to previous
prejudices.

Improving Program Efficiency. The same procedures
could be used to compare the benefits and costs of

Table 5-2

Benefit-Cost or Cost-Effectiveness Ratio

Criteria of Success	Program A	Program B	Program C
Increased social satisfaction	3.0/$1000	2.0/$1000	1.0/$1000
Increased life expectancy	1 year/ $1000	2 years/ $1000	3 years/ $1000
Increased earnings	2.0	2.0	2.0

various medical interventions or approaches used by a particular program in order to determine the most efficient combinations of procedures. The multivariate analysis proposed earlier includes the effects of the presence, the duration, and the quality of program services on each of the measures of success and cost.

There may be a procedure which has no benefit-cost ratio greater than one and no positive cost-effectiveness ratio for any of the possible criteria. Such a procedure probably should be dropped. In some cases, however, procedures have to be treated as complementary sets. For example, diagnostic testing by itself will make no improvement in the individual's behavior; without it useful treatment, however, may be extremely difficult. It is more likely, however, that procedures will vary in their effectiveness, depending on the criterion of success. Once more, a tabular listing for each procedure can be made, including the benefit-cost or cost-effectiveness ratio for each of the criteria in order to facilitate the choice between procedures.

Matching Clients and Health Programs. Finally, the same method of analysis and presentation may be used to identify the effects of various programs and procedures on different types of clients to determine the best combinations for particular groups of potential clients. The multivariate analysis would show whether health procedures produce differential success or costs, depending on the types of clients. From these data, benefit-cost and cost-effectiveness ratios for a particular group of clients could be calculated for all programs and procedures. Once more, the weighting of tabularly presented values will allow cross-program and cross-procedure comparisons.

Steps for Evaluating the Impact of Health Programs: A Summary

In our opinion the impact of all health programs, procedures, technologies, and interventions should be systematically evaluated with such evaluations beginning as soon as each program/procedure becomes operational and continuing on a periodic basis. The preceding discussion provides what may appear to be a confusing number of alternative approaches to measure the impacts and costs of health programs. Here we wish to compress that discussion and to outline what we feel would be a useful procedure for measuring program impact. The steps include the following:

1. Define exactly what comprises the health program, then examine the services, clients and operating conditions of the program.
   a. Determine what is the nature of the program, and how large it is, and with what other programs, procedures, or services is it comparable.
   b. Identify the program's clients and the manner in which they are recruited and selected.
   c. Identify the program staff and the sources and nature of program support.
2. Determine the possible impacts of the program.
   a. Determine the goals of the program as perceived by the commissioners of the evaluation.
   b. Determine the goals of "significant others" who may make use of the evaluation--program administrators, grant

recipients, policy makers who originate or review such programs, other evaluators (possibly through publications), and program clients.
  c. Review evaluations of similar programs, procedures or services to determine the impact measures used and especially those which were significant.
  d. Think of all other possible impacts.
  e. Identify the impacts with the party being affected--society, government (or a particular unit of government), medical professionals, clients, and clients' families.
3. Establish one or more measures of each impact.
  a. Use existing scales and instruments when possible.
  b. Convert health benefits into monetary values based on life expectancy, willingness to pay, or other rationale relative to health benefits wherever possible.
  c. Be concerned with the validity of the measures.
4. Determine which impacts should be measured.
  a. Follow the principle that it is better to measure too many impacts than to omit one which is important, noting that priorities for programs and services change with economic conditions and policy maker preferences.
  b. Eliminate only those impacts which are immeasurable, which will cost too much to measure, or where no significant effect is anticipated.
5. Establish a measurement design which will have internal and external validity in estimating the net impacts of the program.
  a. Note the threats to internal and external validity.
  b. If at all possible, opt for random assignment to control and experimental groups since this provides for internal validity. Make the case for random assignment as strongly as is possible.

     c. If random assignment is ruled out, the next best alternative as far as internal validity is concerned is probably the regression discontinuity design. This design is less useful for generalizing.

     d. If a nonequivalent comparison group is used, note the possible threats to internal validity and realize that the superiority of one group is likely to influence the direction and magnitude of the findings. State the expected biases.

6. Determine the potential costs of the program.

     a. Avoid the use of budget line expenditures as the sole measure of costs.

     b. Apply the concept of opportunity cost to measure benefits foregone due to the existence of the program.

     c. Use marginal productivity theory to aid in the estimation of society's opportunity costs.

     d. Identify the party bearing each of the costs--society, government (or particular units of government), health professionals, clients, and the clients' families.

7. Apply a design which measures the net increment in costs.

     a. Comparisons of clients and control groups should yield estimates of opportunity costs for clients and production lost by society.

     b. Governmental costs should include the services provided to clients and control group members to estimate the net difference.

8. Design procedures for gathering data and analysis.

     a. Determine the appropriate sample size consistent with the variation in the data and level of confidence desired.

     b. Allocate the sample selection among projects or services of differing types and sizes. Impact and cost data should be collected from different-sized programs, if possible, to allow measurement of marginal impacts and costs.

c. Study the strengths and weaknesses of alternative data sources and data gathering techniques, noting that they and the sample size must conform to available funds. Wherever possible rely on an existing data source rather than establishing new data collection procedures. If the evaluation involves contacting persons after the program, efforts should be made to keep track of the individuals so their location is known if they move.

d. Data to be used to measure impacts should be collected at least one year following the program.

e. Cost data should be collected after projects have become fully operable to avoid initial high average costs due to program start-up.

f. During the project, records should be maintained on the nature, length, and cost of all services performed for each participant.

g. Records should also be kept for each person indicating changes in his or her knowledge of health care and preventive services, overall health, and satisfaction with the health services. For each person who drops out of the treatment, an exit interview should be conducted to determine the reasons for leaving the project.

h. Impact and cost data should be identified with individuals so that separate calculations of program effectiveness can be made for different groups of potential clients.

i. Use multivariate analysis to adjust for differences between the control or comparison group members and the participants. Calculate the degree of success on each criterion for the total program, for groups of participants in the program, for various program services, for the care provided by various health professionals, and for various conditions under which the program operates.

9. Adjust the impacts and costs.
   a. Project the impacts for their expected duration and include any expected growth or decline in them.
   b. Discount the impacts and costs to find their present value.
   c. Estimate the effects of externalities and secondary impacts.
   d. Estimate the influence of threats to validity in the evaluation design.

10. Make calculations and discuss the findings.
   a. Present marginal cost-effectiveness or benefit-cost measures (benefit-cost ratio, net present value, and internal rate of return) for each impact under consideration so that the reader can aggregate impacts using his or her own weights.
   b. Aggregate impacts if agreement has been reached on a preference function.
   c. Present separate calculations for significant groups of clients, for different combinations of program services, and for projects operating under differing conditions.
   d. Indicate how these calculations are subject to the assumptions made in the estimation process.
   e. Present your best estimate for the effectiveness of the program.
   f. Suggest any improvements in program efficiency which are derived from the

analysis.[63]

Limitations on Evaluation Techniques

There are three basic limitations on the impact evaluation methods we have presented which should always be kept in mind. First, the analysis will be based only on some of the criteria of success and only on some of the costs of health programs. Our lists of impacts and costs are admittedly incomplete. Even if more were added to each list, constraints on time, funds, and ability would limit the materials which could be considered and important criteria might be omitted. More importantly, however, we consider only those criteria of success and costs which can be measured; ignored are those which cannot be measured. For these reasons the judgments which are made about programs, services, and clients may not always be "right."

Second, even for measureable criteria, correct evaluations of health programs cannot always be designed. We have argued that random assignment to experimental and control groups will permit

---

[63]The Office of Technology Assessment similarly published what they term as ten principles of cost effectiveness analysis and cost benefit analysis methodology (132). Nearly all the principles outlined in this report are included in our approach. We also wish to point out that while interpreting the costs and benefits of health programs, ethical issues need to be discussed which may directly impact on costs. Whether or not to advocate abortion as a method of birth control, or use particular types of life support methodologies for the terminally ill will bear directly on both the costs and benefits of health programs. The assumptions and principles advocated by the health program effects should, consequently, be clearly stated and placed in appropriate perspective relative to the rest of the analysis as pointed out above.

considerably more accurate and trustworthy evaluations than will other methods of sample selection. There are still threats to external validity involved, however, which may limit the generalizability of the findings. Not all variables which could conceivably influence the outcomes and costs of health programs can be included in any analysis. Therefore, an observed relationship may be due to some other factor which is correlated with the two variables being examined. For example, it may be found that an anti-smoking campaign is associated with lower levels of lung cancer than a program of industrial pollution controls. If, however, local air quality is not a variable in the analysis, and the two programs occurred in Tucson, a different relationship might be found if the antismoking campaign and pollution control program were tried in Los Angeles. Likewise, we measure relationships which exist for a given period of time. They may change over time as other unanalyzed variables change. Thus, while the ratios obtained from the type of analyses may be accurate for the group under study, they may be difficult to generalize.

The third limitation has been discussed before. The estimates of benefits and costs are usually averages for the health programs and services. They do not measure directly the effect of changes in program size. While one program may have considerably higher average ratios than another, increasing the size of that program or service may lead to smaller gains in success per dollar of cost than would occur by increasing the program with the lower average ratios. Until further information is available on marginal gains and costs, we can only assume that the effects of changing the size of programs or services will be directly related to their ratios of average success to costs.

Finally, there is a problem which this primer hopes to solve. Evaluations to date have been on a program by program basis, each using different methodologies. Typically, each study uses a different type of control or comparison group and a different way of handling externalities and secondary effects. Data sources, types of questions, and measures of benefits will differ with each study. Different periods will be used for projecting benefits and different discount rates will be employed for estimating present values. There will be similar differences in the techniques for cost measurement. In order to make the results of the studies comparable, all of the assumptions and techniques need to be equated. It is our hope that if evaluators follow the ideas and procedures presented in this primer, there will be sufficient similarity among individual studies to make the comparable. [64]

A Final Word for Impact Evaluation

The type of analysis we have proposed is difficult to conduct and obviously filled with pitfalls. It may not be correct when completed. There are reasons for its use, however. It forces those responsible for health program decisions to attach weights to their goals and to quantify the success and costs of a program as far as is possible rather than rest content with vague qualitative judgments and personal hunches. This is obviously a good thing in itself; some information is better than none. Also, it has the very valuable byproduct of raising questions which would otherwise not have been asked. There is a considerable expansion in the outlook with which the programs are viewed; from daily operational questions to the broader perspectives of social impacts and costs. Thus, even though impact evaluation may not always give the "right" answers, it may lead to the

---

[64]The best alterantive appears to be to conduct multiprogram evaluations where a conscious effort is made to evaluate more than one program using the same techniques, assumptions, time period, and so forth. While methodologically this procedure is preferred, the simultaneous evaluation of a number of programs requires considerable resources, and administering such a project becomes a major job which may flounder due to its complexities.

asking of more "right" questions if used sensibly. As experience and expertise are accumulated, this method should lead to better answers.

Exercise 5-1

Mobile coronary care units of Horizon City are presumed to have cut prehospital deaths in half; survivors have been judged to have a prognosis comparable to past heart attack survivors. The local health planning agency estimates that while prior to the installation of the mobile coronary care units there were 150 prehospital deaths per year, there are only 75 now. The costs for the units amounted to $80,000 for the first year, $60,000 for the second year, and $50,000 per year for the succeeding years. Discounting costs at 5%, 10%, and 15%, estimate the cost savings for clients and the community of having the mobile coronary unit available for the next 20 years. Specify the method used for estimating the valuation of life, and the reason for choosing it. Indicate any further issues the community or government needs to consider in determining whether or not to continue support of the program at Horizon City.

Exercise 5-2

Discuss the rationale underlying the steps outlined in this volume for evaluating the impact of health programs. Select a health program in your community and demonstrate how each of these steps may be applied to arrive at a systematic evaluation of the program.

Suggested Readings

Altman, S. and Socholitzky, E. "The Cost of Ambulatory Care in Alternative Settings: A Review of Major Research Findings," Annual Review of Public Health 2, 1981.

Cretin, S. "Cost-Benefit Analysis of Treatment and Prevention of Myocardial Infarction," Health Services Research 12, Summer 1977.

Klarman, H., et al. "Cost-Effectiveness Analysis Applied to the Treatment of Chronic Renal Disease," Medical Care 6, January-February 1968.

Luft, H. "Benefit-Cost Analysis and Public Polity Implementation: From Normative to Positive Analysis," Public Policy 24, Fall 1976.

Schoenbaum, S., et al. "The Swine-Influenza Decision," New England Journal of Medicine, 295, September 30, 1976.

Stange, P. and Sumner, A. "Predicting Treatment Costs and Life Expectancy for End-Stage Renal Disease," New England Journal of Medicine 298, February 16, 1978.

Weinstein, M.C., and Stason, W. "Foundations of Cost-Effectiveness Analysis for Health and Medical Practices," New England Journal of Medicine 296, March 31, 1977.

1. Acton, J. Evaluating Public Programs to Save
    Lives: The Case of Heart Attacks, Santa Monica,
    California: Rand Corporation, 1973.

2. Akpon, C.A., Katz, S. and Densen, P.M. "Methods
    of Classifying Disability and Severity of Ill-
    ness in Ambulatory Care Patients," Medical Care,
    (Supplement) 11, 1973.

3. Albritton, R. "Cost-Benefits of Measles Eradi-
    cation: Effects of a Federal Intervention,"
    Political Annals 4, Winter 1978.

4. Altman, S. and Blandon, R., eds. Medical Tech-
    nology: The Culprit Behind Health Care Costs?
    proceedings of the Sun Valley Forum on National
    Health, DHHEW publication No. (PHS) 79-3216,
    Washington, D.C.: U.S. Government Printing
    Office, August 1977.

5. Altman, S. and Socholitzky, E. "The Cost of
    Ambulatory Care in Alternative Settings: A
    Review of Major Research Findings," Annual
    Review of Public Health 2, 1981.

6. Attkisson, C., Hargreaves, W.A. and Horowitz,
    M.J., eds. Evaluation of Human Service Pro-
    grams, New York: Academic Press, 1978.

7. Averill, R., et al. "A Cost-Benefit Analysis of
    Continued Stay Certification," Medical Care 15,
    February 1977.

8. Avery, A.D., et al. Quality of Medical Care
    Assessment Using Outcome Measures: Eight Di-
    sease-Specific Applications, Rand Note R-
    2021/2/HEW, Santa Monica, California: Rand,
    August 1976.

9. Backhaut, B. "Refining Cost Benefit Estimates
    of Methadone Programs," National Conference
    Methadone Treatment Proceedings 2, 1973.

10. Balinsky, W. and Berger, R. "A Review of the
     Research on General Health Status Indexes, "
     Medical Care, 13, 1975.

11. Barrett, T., et al. "Making Evaluation Systems
     Cost-Effective," Hospital Community Psychology
     3, March 1977.

12. Bay, K., et al. "The Worth of a Screening
     Program: An Application of a Statistical De-
     cision Model for the Benefit Evaluation of
     Screening Projects," American Journal of Public
     Health 66, February 1976.

13. Berg, R.L. "Establishing the Values of Various
     Conditions of Life for a Health Status Index,"
     Health Status Indexes, R.L. Berg, ed.,
     Chicago: Hospital Research and Educational
     Trust, 1973.

14. Berry, E., et al. The Economic Cost of Alcohol
     Abuse and Alcoholism, 1971, Policy Analysis,
     Inc., Boston, 1974, HWM 42-73-114(NIA).

15. Blumstein, A. and Cassidy, R. "Benefit-Cost
     Analysis of Family Planning," Socio-Econmic
     Plan. Science 7, 1973.

16. Boggs, D. "Applying the Techniques of Cost
     Effectiveness to the Delivery of Dental Ser-
     vices," Journal of Public Health Dentistry 33,
     Fall 1973.

17. Boissoneau, R. "Point of View: Cost Effective-
     ness in the Health Care System," Journal of
     American Dietitic Association 66, May 1975.

18. Bonjean, C.M., Jill, R.J. and McLennore, S.D.,
     eds. Sociological Measurement: An Inventory of
     Scales and Indices, San Francisco: Chandler,
     1967.

19. Boruch, R.F.   "On Common Contentions About
     Randomized Field Experiments," in *Evaluation
     Studies Review Annual*, G.V. Blass, ed., Vol.
     1. Beverly Hills: Sage Publications, 1976.

20. Boruch, R.F. and Riecken, H.W., eds. *Social
     Experimentation, A Method for Planning and
     Evaluating Social Intervention*, New York:
     Academic Press, 1975.

21. Borus, M.E., ed.   *Evaluating the Impact of
     Manpower Programs*, Lexington: D.C. Heath and
     Co., 1972.

22. Brock, R.H.   "Quality Assurance Today and To-
     morrow: Forecast for the Future," *Annals of
     Internal Medicine* 85 (6), December 1976.

23. Brock, R.H.   "Quality of Care Assessment:
     Policy Relevant Issues," *Policy Sciences*, Sep-
     tember 1974.

24. Brock, R.H. and Avery, A.D.   *Quality Assurance
     Mechanisms in the United States: From There to
     Where?* Rand Note P-5520, Santa Monica, Cali-
     fornia: Rand, October, 1975.

25. Brown, J.   "Reducing the Cost of Medical Care:
     Prevention as a Cost Effective Measure," *Texas
     Medicine* 75, March 1979.

26. Bryers, E. and Hawthorne, J.   "Screening for
     Mild Hypertension: Costs and Benefits," *Journal
     of Epidemology and Community Health* 32, Septem-
     ber 1978.

27. Bunker, J.P., ed. *Costs, Risks, and Benefits of
     Surgery*, New York: Oxford University Press,
     1977.

28. Bush, J., et al. "Cost-Effectiveness Using a Health Status Index: Analysis of the New York State PKU Screening Program," in Health Status Indexes: Proceedings of a Conference, R.L. Berg, ed., Chicago: Hospital Research and Educational Trust, 1973.

29. Bush, J.W., Chen, M.N. and Patrick, D.L. "Social Indications for Health Based on Functional Status and Prognosis," in Proceedings of the Social Statistics Section, American Statistical Association, Washington, D.C., 1972.

30. Cain, G. "Regression and Selection Models to Improve Nonexperimental Claims," in Evaluation and Experiment: Some Critical Issues in Assessing Social Programs, C.A. Bennett and A.A. Lumsdaine, eds., New York: Academic Press, 1975.

31. Campbell, D.T. "Reforms as Experiments," in Handbook of Evaluation Research, E. Struening and M. Guttentag, eds., Vol. 1, Beverly Hills: Sage Publications, 1975.

32. Campbell, T. and Boruch, R.F. "Making the Case for Randomized Assignment to Treatments by Considering the Alternatives: Six Ways in Which Quasi-Experimental Evaluations in Compensatory Education Tend to Underestimate Effect," in Evaluation and Experiment: Some Critical Issues in Assessing Social Programs, C.A. Bennett and A.A. Lumsdaine, eds., New York: Academic Press, 1975.

33. Campbell, D.T. and Stanley, J.C. Experimental and Quasi-Experimental Designs for Research, Chicago: Rand McNally and Co., 1971.

34. Catford, J. and Fowkes, F. "Economic Benefits of Day Care Abortion," Community Medicine 1, May 1979.

35.   Chawla, M. and Steinhardt, B. "Episode of Care Accounting Methodology for a Cost-Effectiveness Approach to Quality Assurance in a HMO," PHS-HMS-110-73-402, Bethesda, Md.: Public Health Service, May 1975.

36.   Christoffel, J.D. and Loventhal, M. "Evaluating the Quality of Ambulatory Health Care: A Review of Emerging Methods," Medical Care 15 (11), November 1977.

37.   Cochrane, A. Effectiveness and Efficiency: Random Reflections on Health Services, London: Burgess & Son Ltd., Nuffield Provincial Hospitals Trust, 1972.

38.   Cochrane, A. "Issues in Benefit-Cost Analyses of the Vocational Rehabilitation Program," American Rehabilitation 1, November-December 1975.

39.   Cochrane, A. "Mental Retardation: An Economist's Approach," Mental Retardation 14, December 1976.

40.   Cochrane, A., et al. Benefit-Cost Analysis for Mental Retardation Programs, Theoretical Considerations and a Model for Application, Ann Arbor: University of Michigan, Institute for the Study of Mental Retardation and Related Disabilities, 1971.

41.   Cochrane, A., et al. "Cost Analysis of a Multiphasic Screening Program," New England Journal of Medicine 280, May 8, 1969.

42.   Committee on Vital and Health Statistics, Publication No. (PMS) 80-1157, April 1980.

43.   Congress of the United States, Office of Tech-
       nology Assessment, Assessing the Efficacy and
       Safety of Medical Technologies, Washington,
       D.C.:   U.S. Government Printing Office, Septem-
       ber 1978.

44.   Congress of the United States, Office of Tech-
       nology Assessment, The Implications of Cost
       Effectiveness Analysis of Medical Technology,
       "Background Paper #1: Methodological Issues and
       Literature Review," September 1980.

45.   Congress of the United States, Office of Tech-
       nology Assessment, The Implications of Cost-
       Effectiveness Analysis of Medical Technology,
       Appendix D, "Values Ethics, and CBA in Health
       Care," August 1980.

46.   Cook, T.D. and Campbell D.T. Quasi-Experimenta-
       tion Designs and Analysis Issues for Field
       Settings, New York: Rand McNally, 1979.

47.   Cook, T.D. and Gruder, C.L. "Metaevaluation Re-
       search," Evaluation Quarterly 2, 1978.

48.   Cook, T.D. and Reichardts, C.S., eds. Qualita-
       tive and Quantitative Methods in Evaluation
       Research, Beverly Hills: Sage Publications,
       1979.

49.   Cooper, B.S. and Rice, D.P. "The Economic Cost
       of Illness Revisited," Social Security Bulletin,
       February 1976.

50.   "Cost-Effectiveness Studies," British Medical
       Journal 2, September 23, 1978.

51.   Cretin, S. "Cost-Benefit Analysis of Treatment
       and Prevention of Myocardial Infarction," Health
       Services Research 12, Summer 1977.

52.   Cruze, A.M., et al. _The Economic Cost to_
      Society of Alcohol, Drug Abuse, and Mental
      Illness, ADAMHA, Contract No. 283-79-001, Re-
      search Triangle Institute, September 1981.

53.   Crystal, R. and Brewster, A. "Cost-Benefit and
      Cost-Effectiveness Analyses in the Health
      Field: An Introduction," _Inquiry_ 3, 1966.

54.   Doherty, N., et al. "Cost-Effectiveness Anal-
      ysis and Alternative Health Care Programs for
      the Elderly," _Health Service Research_ 12, Summer
      1977.

55.   Doherty, N. and Powell, E. "Effects of Age and
      Years of Exposure on the Economic Benefits of
      Fluoridation," _Journal of Dental Research_ 53,
      August 1974.

56.   Donabedian, A. "Evaluating the Quality of
      Medical Care," _Milbank Memorial Fund Quarterly_,
      (Part 2) 44, 1966.

57.   Drummond, M.F. _Principles of Economic Appraisal_
      in Health Care, Oxford University Press, 1972.

58.   Dunlop, D. "Benefit-Cost Analysis: A Review of
      Its Applicability in Policy Analysis for
      Delivering Health Services," _Society of Scien-_
      tific Medicine 9, March 1975.

59.   Edwards, D.W., Yarris, R.M. and Mueller, D.P.
      "Does Patient Satisfaction Correlate with Suc-
      cess?" _Hospital and Community Psychiatry_ 29
      (3), March 1978.

60.   Farber, M. and Finkelstein, S. "A Cost-Benefit
      Analysis of a Mandatory Premarital Rubella-
      Antibody Screening Program, _New England Journal_
      of Medicine 300, April 1978.

61. Farshal, S. and Bush, J.W. "A Health Status
     Index and Its Application to Health Services
     Outcomes," Operations Research 18(6), November-
     December 1970.

62. Fein, R. "But On the Other Hand: High Blood
     Pressure, Economics and Equity," New England
     Journal of Medicine 296, March 31, 1977.

63. Fein, R. "On Measuring Economic Benefits of
     Health Probrams," in Ethics and Health Policy,
     R. Veatch and R. Branson, eds., Cambridge,
     Mass.: Ballinger, 1976.

64. Fein, R., et al. "Cost-Benefit Analysis and the
     Evaluation of Psychiatric Services," Psycholog-
     ical Medicine 7, November 1977.

65. Ferman, L.A. "Some Perspectives on Evaluating
     Social Welfare Programs, The Annals of the
     American Academy of Political and Social Science
     385, September 1969.

66. Fitzgerald, N.M., Hormuth, S.E. and Cook, T.D.
     "Quasi-Experimental Methods in Community Psy-
     chology Research," in Knowledge Building in
     Community Psychology, E.C. Suskind and D.C.
     Klein, eds., New York: Holt, Rinehart, and
     Winston, 1981.

67. Georgetown University, Public Services Labor-
     atory. Bibliography on the Social and Economic
     Costs of Illness, a report to the National
     Institutes of Health under Contract NO1-OD-5-
     2121.

68. Goldschmidt, P. "A Cost-Effectiveness Model for
     Evaluating Health Care Programs: Application to
     Drug Abuse Treatment," Inquiry 13, March 1976.

69.   Goldschmidt, P.   "Cost-Benefit Analysis of
       Health Services, Annals of the American Academy
       of Political and Social Science 399, January
       1972.

70.   Goldschmidt, P.   "Toward Cost-Benefit Evalua-
       tions of Health Education, Some Concepts,
       Methods, and Examples," Health Education Mono-
       graph 2, 1974.

71.   Gonnella, J.S., Louis, D.Z. and McCord, J.J.
       "The Staging Concept--An Approach to the Assess-
       ment of Outcome of Ambulatory Care," Medical
       Care, Supplement 17 (5), May 1979.

72.   Grosse, R.   "Cost-Benefit Analysis of Health
       Services," Annals of the American Academy of
       Political and Social Science 399, January 1972.

73.   Guerney, B.G., Jr.   Relationship Enhancement:
       Skill-Training Program for Therapy, Problem-
       Prevention and Enrichment, San Francisco:
       Jossey-Bass, 1977.

74.   Guillette, W., et al. "Day Hospitalization as a
       Cost Effective Alternative to Inpatient Care: A
       Pilot Study," Hospital Community Psychiatry 29,
       August 1978.

75.   Hannan, T. "The Benefits and Costs of Methadone
       Maintenance," Public Policy 24, Spring 1976.

76.   "Health Status Indexes, Work in Progress," 2
       (4), Health Services Research, Winter, 1976.

77.   Heckman, J.J.   "The Common Structure of Statis-
       tical Models of Truncation, Sample Selection,
       and Limited Dependent Variables and a Simple
       Estimator for Such Models," Annals of Economic
       and Social Measurement 5 (4), Fall 1976.

78. Hellinger, F.J. "Cost-Benefit Analysis of Health Care: Past Applications and Future Prospects," Inquiry 3, Bulletin 250, Fall 1980.

79. Hertzman, M., et al. "Cost-Benefit Analysis and Alcoholism," Journal of the Study of Alcohol 38, July 1977.

80. Hodgson, T. and Meiners, M. Guidelines for Cost of Illness Studies in the Public Health Service, for the PHS Task Force on Cost of Illness Studies, Washington, D.C.: HHS, May 31, 1979.

81. Holahan, J. The Economics of Drug Addiction and Control in Washington, D.C.: A Model for Estimation of Costs and Benefits of Rehabilitation, Washington, D.C.: District of Columbia Department of Corrections, 1970.

82. Holahan, J. "Measuring Benefits From Alternative Heroin Policies," in National Conference on Methadone Treatment Proceedings 2, 1973.

83. Jackson, S. and Ward, D. "Prevention of Institutionalization: A Cost-Effectiveness Model of Community Based Alternatives," presented at the Annual Meeting of the American Public Health Association, Miami Beach, Fla., Oct. 17-21, 1976.

84. Jaffe, F., et al. "Short-Term Benefits and Costs of U.S. Family Planning Programs, 1970-1975," Family Planning Perspectives 9, March-April 1977.

85. Joglekar, P. "Cost-Benefit Studies of Health Care Programs: Choosing Methods for Desired Results," paper presented at the Joint National Meeting of TIMS/ORSA, Washington, D.C., May 1980.

86. Jong, A., and Gluck, G. "Factors Influencing
     the Cost-Effectiveness of Community Health
     Center Dental Programs in the USA," Community
     Dentistry and Oral Epidemiology 2, 1974.

87. JWK International. Benefit-Cost Analysis of
     Alcoholism Treatment Centers, Contract No. ADM-
     281-75-0031, Annandale, Virginia: May 4, 1976.

88. Kane, R.L., et al. "Measuring Outcomes of Care
     in An Ambulatory Primary Care Population,"
     Journal of Community Health 1 (4), Summer 1976.

89. Kirby, W.   "Cost-Benefit Analysis in a Large
     Health Care System," in Cost-Benefit Analysis,
     M. Kendall, ed., New York: American Elsevier,
     1971.

90. Klarman, H., "Applications of Cost-Benefit
     Analysis to the Health Services and the Special
     Case of Technologic Innovation," International
     Journal of Health Service 4, Spring 1974.

91. Klarman, H.   "Present Status of Cost-Benefit
     Analysis in the Health Field, American Journal
     of Public Health 57, November 1967.

92. Klarman, H., et al.   "Cost-Effectiveness Anal-
     ysis Applied to the Treatment of Chronic Renal
     Disease," Medical Care 6, January-February 1968.

93. Kristein, M.   "Cost-Effectiveness Analysis for
     HSA Planning," paper presented at the Annual
     Meeting of the American Public Health Associa-
     tion, New York, NY, November 7, 1979.

94. Kristein, M.   "Economic Issues in Prevention,"
     Preventative Medicine 6, 1977.

95. Lave, J. and Lave, L. "Measuring the Effective-
     ness of Prevention," Milbank Memorial Fund
     Quarterly 55, 1977.

96. Layard, R., ed. Cost-Benefit Analysis, Middle-
     sex, England: Penguin Books, 1977.

97. Luce, B. "Allocating Costs and Benefits in
     Disease Prevention Programs: An Application to
     Cervical Cancer Screening," in The Implications
     of Cost-Effectiveness Analysis of Medical Tech-
     nology, "Background Paper #2: Case Studies of
     Medical Technologies," prepared at the Office of
     Technology Assessment, U.S. Congress, Washing-
     ton, D.C.: 1980.

98. Luft, H. "Benefit-Cost Analysis and Public
     Policy Implementation: From Normative to Pos-
     itive Analysis," Public Policy 24, Fall 1976.

99. Luft, H. "Cost-Efficiency of the Mental Health
     Delivery System: A Review of the Literature on
     Hospital Care," American Journal of Public
     Health 60, November 1970.

100. Luft, H. and Cotton, J. "The Cost of Mental
     Health Care Under Changing Treatment Methods:
     One Criterion Out of Many," International Jour-
     nal of Psychology 4, August 1967.

101. Luft, H. and Lewicki, A. "What Do We Gain From
     the Sixth Stool Guaiac?," New England Journal of
     Medicine 292, July 31, 1975.

102, McKillop, W. "Assessing Quality of Medical
     Care," Hospital Administration, Fall 1974.

103. Mishan, E.J. Cost Benefit Analysis, Washington,
     D.C.: Praeger Publication, 1976.

104. Murnaghn, J. "Health Indicators and Information
     Systems for the Year 2000," Annual Review of
     Public Health 2, 1981.

105. Mushkin, S. "Knowledge and Choices in Health: Cost-Benefit Analysis in Health Policy Assessments," Washington, D.C., Georgetown University, Public Services Laboratory, 1977.

106. National Center for Health Statistics. Catalog of Publications of the National Center for Health Statistics. DHHS Publication No. (PHS) 8-1301, Washington, D.C.: July 1980.

107. National Center for Health Statistics. Catalog of Public Use Data Tapes, DHHS No. (PHS) 81-1213, November 1980.

108. Neuhauser, D. and Lewicki, A. "What Do We Gain from the Sixth Stool Guaiac?" New England Journal of Medicine 293, July 31, 1975.

109. Phelps, C. "Benefit/Cost Assessment for Quality Assurance Program," Rand Corporation Report R-1954-HEW, Santa Monica: Rand Corporation, 1976.

110. Pole, J. "The Cost-Effectiveness of Screening," Proceedings of the Royal Society of Medicine 65, December 1971.

111. Prest, A.R. and Turvey, R. "Cost-Benefit Analysis: A Survey," in Surveys of Economic Theory, Vol. III, New York: St. Martin's Press, 1967.

112. Rice, D. and Cooper, B.S. "The Economic Value of Human Life," American Journal of Public Health 57, November 1967.

113. Riechen, H.W. and Boruch, R.F., eds. Social Experimentation, New York: Academic Press, 1974.

114. Robinson, J.P. , Rusk, J. and Head, K. Measures of Political Attitudes, Ann Arbor: Institute for Social Research, University of Michigan, 1969.

115. Robinson, J. and Shaver, P. Measures of Social Psychological Attitudes, Ann Arbor: Institute for Social Research, University of Michigan, 1973.

116. Rowe, D. and Bisbee, J. "Preventive Health Care in the HMO: Cost-Benefit Issues," Journal of the American College Health Associations 26 (6), June 1978.

117. Rutstein, D.D., et al. "Measuring the Quality of Medical Care--A Clinical Method," New England Journal of Medicine 294, March 11, 1976.

118. Salasin, S. "Exploring Goal-Free Evaluation: An Interview with Michael Scriven," Evaluation 2 (1), 1974.

119. Scanlon, J. "Proceedings: Cost Savings/Benefit Analysis of Drug Abuse Treatment," American Journal of Drug and Alcohol Abuse 3, 1976.

120. Schaefer, M. "Demand Versus Need for Medical Services in a General Cost-Benefit Setting," American Journal of Public Health 65, May 1975.

121. Scheffler, R. "A Methodological Framework for Cost-Benefit Analysis in Health," in Evaluation in Health Services Delivery, proceedings of an Engineering Foundation Conference, South Berwick, Maine, Aug. 19-24, 1973.

122. Scheffler, R. and Rovin, S. "Periodontal Disease: Assessing the Effectiveness and Costs of the Keyes Technique," in The Implications of Cost-Effectiveness Analysis of Medical Technology, "Background Paper #2: Case Studies of Medical Technologies," Washington, D.C.: Office of Technology Assessment, U.S. Congress, 1980.

123. Schoenbaum, S., et al. "The Swine-Influenza Decision," New England Journal of Medicine 295, September 30, 1976.

124. Schroeder, S.A. and Donaldson, M.S. "The Feasi-
     bility of an Outcome Approach to Quality Assur-
     ance--A Report from One HMO," Medical Care 14
     (1), January 1976.

125. Schulberg, H.C. Program Evaluation in the
     Health Fields, New York: Behavioral Publica-
     tions, Inc., 1969.

126. Scriven, M. "Pros and Cons About Goal-Free
     Evaluation," The Journal of Educational Evalua-
     tion 3 (4), December 1972.

127. Shapiro, S. "End Result Measurement of Medical
     Care," Milbank Memorial Fund Quarterly 45, 1967.

128. Shelton, J., Hollister, L. and Gorka, E. "Quan-
     tifying Alcoholic Impairment," Modern Medicine,
     November 17, 1969.

129. Shepard, D.S. and Thompson, M.S. "Cost
     Effectiveness Analysis in Health," Group Prac-
     tice Journal 30 (2), Fall 1981.

130. Smith, R.E. "The Opportunity Cost of Partici-
     pating in a Training Program," Journal of Human
     Resources 6 (4), Fall 1971.

131. Stahler, G. and Tash, W.R., eds. Innovative Ap-
     proaches in Mental Health Program Evaluation,
     New York: Academic Press, 1982.

132. Stange, P. "The Feasibility of Economic Eval-
     uation of Diagnostic Procedures: The Case of CT
     Scanning," in The Implications of Cost-
     Effectiveness Analysis of Medical Technology,
     "Background Paper #2: Case Studies of Medical
     Technologies," Washington, D.C.: Office of
     Technology Assessment, U.S. Congress, 1980.

133. Stange, P., et al. "The Application of Economic
     Analysis to Evaluation of Alcoholism Rehabili-
     tation Programs," Inquiry 14, March 1977.

134. Stange, P. and Gish, O. "Mobile Health Ser-
      vices: A Study in Cost-Effectiveness," Medical
      Care 15, April 1977.

135. Stange, P. and Sumner A. "Predicting Treatment
      Costs and Life Expectancy for End-Stage Renal
      Disease," New England Journal of Medicine 298,
      February 16, 1978.

136. Stange, P. and Weinstein, M. "Allocation of
      Resources to Manage Hypertension," New England
      Journal of Medicine 296, March 31, 1977.

137. Starfield, B. "Measurement of Outcome: A
      Proposed Scheme," Milbank Memorial Fund Quar-
      terly (Health and Society) 52, Winter 1974.

138. Struening, E. and Guttentag, M., eds. Handbook
      of Evaluation Research, Vol. 1, Beverly Hills:
      Sage Publications, 1975.

139. Suits, D.B. Statistics: An Introduction to
      Quantitative Economic Research, Chicago: Rand
      McNally & Co., 1971.

140. Thompson, H.C. and Osborne, C.E. "Office Re-
      cords in the Evaluation of Quality of Care,"
      Medical Care 14 (4), April 1976.

141. Towery, O.B., Seidenberg, G.R. and Santoro, V.
      Quality Assurance for Alcohol, Drug Abuse, and
      Mental Health Services: An Annotated Biblio-
      graphy, Rockville, Maryland: ADAMHA, 1979.

142. U.S. Department of Health, Education, and Wel-
      fare, Disease Control Programs: Arthritis,
      Washington, D.C.: U.S. Government Printing
      Office, 1966.

143. U.S. Department of Health and Human Services,
     Report of the National Committee on Vital and
     Health Statistics, Publication No. (PMS)80-1157,
     Washington, D.C.: April 1980.

144. Veatch, R.M. "Justice and Valuing Lives," in
     Life Span, edited by R.M. Veatch, San Francisco,
     California: Harper and Row, Publishing, 1979.

145. Wainer, K.E. and Hutton, R.C. The Benefit-Costs
     and Cost-Effectiveness Analyses in Health
     Care: A Bibliography, prepared for the Congres-
     sional Office of Technology Assessment under
     Contract No. OTA-C-78-428.

146. Wardell, W. "Assessment of the Benefits, Risks,
     and Costs of Medical Programs," in Benefits and
     Risks in Medical Care, D. Taylor, ed., London:
     White Crescent Press, Ltd., 1974.

147. Ware, J.E. and Johnston, S. Conceptualizationa
     nd Measurement of Health for Adults in the
     Health Insurance Study, Vol. III, Mental Health,
     R-1987/3, Washington, D.C.: 1979.

148. Weinstein, M. "Economic Evaluation of Medical
     Procedures and Technologies: Progress, Pro-
     blems, and Prospects," in Medical Technology,
     proceedings of the Urban Institute Conference,
     National Center for Health Services Research,
     West Palm Beach, Fla., Dec. 10-12, 1978.

149. Weinstein, M., et al. "An Alternative to Mental
     Hospital Treatment: III. Economic Benefit-Cost
     Analysis," unpublished paper, Madison, Wis.,
     December 1978.

150. Weinstein, M. and Stason, W. "Economic Consid-
     erations in the Management of Mild Hyper-
     tension," Annals of the N.Y. Academy of Sciences
     304, March 30, 1976.

151. Weinstein, M. and Stason, W. "Foundations of Cost-Effectiveness Analysis for Health and Medical Practices," New England Journal of Medicine 296, March 31, 1977.

152. Weinstein, M. and Stason, W. Hypertension: A Policy Perspective, Cambridge, Mass.: Harvard University Press, 1976.

153. Weiss, C.H. "Interviewing in Evaluation Research," in Handbook of Evaluation Research, E.L. Struening and M. Guttentag, Eds., Vol. 1, Beverly Hills: Sage Publications, 1975.

154. Wholey, J.S., et al. Federal Evaluation Policy: Analyzing the Effects of Public Programs, Washington, D.C.: The Urban Institute, 1970.

155. Williamson, J.W. "Evaluating the Quality of Patient Care, A Strategy Relating Outcome and Process Assessment," Journal of the American Medical Association 218, 1971.

156. Williamson, J.W., et al. "Health Accounting: An Outcome-Based System of Quality Assurances: Illustrative Application to Hyptertension," Bulletin, New York Academy of Medicine 57, 1975.

157. Wiseman, J. "Cost-Benefit Analysis and Health Service Policy," Scottish Journal of Political Economics 10, February 1963.

158. Witte, J. "The Theory and Practice of Cost-Utility, Cost-Effectiveness, and Cost-Benefit Analysis in Behavioral Medicine: Toward Delivering More Care for Less Money," in A Comprehensive Handbook of Behavioral Medicine, J. Ferguson and B. Taylor, eds., Englewood Cliffs, NJ: Spectrum Publications, Inc., 1979.

159. Witte, J., et al. "The Benefits From 10 Years of Measles Immunization in the United States," Public Health Report 90, May-June 1975.

160. Yates, B. "Cost-Effectiveness Analysis: Using it for Our Own Good," SPAA Newsletter, American Psychological Association 8 (4), May 1977.

161. Zeckhauser, R. and Sheppard, D. "Where Now For Saving Lives?," Law and Contemporary Problems 40 (4), 1976.